# TORAH YOGA

## תורה יוגה

## Experiencing Jewish Wisdom
## Through Classic Postures

### Diane Bloomfield

AN ARTHUR KURZWEIL BOOK

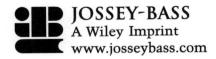

JOSSEY-BASS
A Wiley Imprint
www.josseybass.com

Published by Jossey-Bass
A Wiley Imprint
989 Market Street, San Francisco, CA 94103-1741   www.josseybass.com

Jossey-Bass books and products are available through most bookstores. To contact Jossey-Bass directly
call our Customer Care Department within the U.S. at 800-956-7739, outside the U.S. at 317-572-3986,
or fax 317-572-4002.

Jossey-Bass also publishes its books in a variety of electronic formats. Some content that appears in print
may not be available in electronic books.

Yoga postures photographed by Chris Grey.

The author of this book is not a physician and the ideas, procedures, and suggestions in this book are not
intended as a substitute for the medical advice of a trained health professional. All matters regarding your
health require medical supervision. Consult your physician before adopting the suggestions in this book,
as well as about any condition that may require diagnosis or medical attention. The author and publisher
disclaim any liability arising directly or indirectly from the use of this book.

**Library of Congress Cataloging-in-Publication Data**

Bloomfield, Diane, date.
  Torah yoga: experiencing Jewish wisdom through classic postures / Diane Bloomfield.—1st ed.
    p. cm.
  "An Arthur Kurzweil book."
  Includes bibliographical references.
  ISBN 0–7879–7057–3
  1. Bible. O.T. Pentateuch—Meditations. 2. Yoga. 3. Self-realization—Religious aspects—Judaism. 4.
Spiritual life—Judaism. I. Title.
BS1225.54.B55 2004
296.7'2—dc22                                                                    2003026450

Printed in the United States of America
FIRST EDITION
*PB Printing*          10  9  8  7  6  5  4  3  2  1

# Contents

Acknowledgments                                                vii

Introduction                                                    xi

Using This Book                                                xxi

1   The Hidden Light                                            1
    *Centering Meditation*        7
    *Mountain Posture*        9
    *Triangle Posture*        11
    *Warrior Two Posture*        14
    *Standing Forward Bend*        16
    *Simple Sitting Twist*        19
    *Bridge Posture*        21

2   Constant Renewal                                           23
    *Opening Meditation*        28
    *Seated Mountain Posture*        29
    *Extended Child Posture*        31
    *Downward Dog Posture*        33
    *Locust Posture*        35
    *Cobra Posture*        38

3   Leaving Egypt                                              41
    *Opening Meditation*        47
    *Extended Side Angle Stretch*        48
    *Wide Legs Standing Forward Bend*        50
    *Staff Posture*        53
    *Head Beyond Knee Forward Bend*        55
    *Reclining Mountain Posture*        58
    *Knee-to-Chest Posture*        59

*Reclining Leg Stretch*     61
*Reclining Twist*     64
*Resting with Legs on Chair*     66

**4  The Essential Self**     67
*Opening Meditation*     72
*Chair Twist Posture*     73
*Supported Standing Forward Bend with Chair*     75
*Standing Forward Bend over One Leg*     77
*Revolved Triangle Posture*     80
*Hero Posture*     83
*Resting Fish Posture*     86

**5  Body Prayer and Alignment**     89
*Meet-Your-Spine Meditation*     96
*Upward Reaching Prayer Posture*     97
*Tree Posture*     100
*Warrior One Posture*     103
*Reclining Hero Posture*     105
*Camel Posture*     108
*Bow Posture*     110

**6  Daily Satisfaction**     113
*Centering Meditation*     120
*Cobbler Posture*     121
*Supported Cobbler Posture*     123
*Sitting Forward Bend*     125
*Seated Angle Posture*     128
*Supported Cross-Legged Forward Bend*     132

**7  Remembering to Rest**     133
*Opening Meditation*     141
*Supported Extended Child Posture*     142
*Resting Side Twist*     144
*Supported Fish Posture*     145
*Supported Bridge Posture*     147
*Gentle Inversion Posture*     149
*Relaxation Posture*     151

Glossary     153

Notes     157

Annotated Yoga Bibliography     163

The Author     165

# Acknowledgments

I T IS IRONIC that writing this book, which one might assume to be a solitary endeavor, has brought me more deeply into community with others than ever before. A whole community of people—including family, friends, students, teachers, and colleagues—has showered me with encouragement and love.

*Generosity* is the word that springs to mind when I think about all those who helped me—generosity of time, heart, knowledge, and skill. Thank you, you generous band of angels, for offering me your essential help in so many different ways. I am deeply grateful.

A loving thanks goes to the following people:

My husband, Jonathan, for wholeheartedly devoting his time and talent to this book. His love, belief in me, and constant enthusiasm all provided daily fuel for the task of writing. He was with me discussing, arguing, agonizing, clarifying, reveling, and rejoicing over every thought and every word. There is not one comma or period that he is not intimately aware of. I cannot thank him enough.

Arthur Kurzweil, for believing in me and my work, and in particular for being such a supportive, enthusiastic, and magical midwife in the birth of this book.

Alan Rinzler and Catherine Craddock, of Jossey-Bass, for their clear, respectful, and extremely helpful editing suggestions, as well as for their friendly welcome to the world of publishing.

Iyengar yoga teacher Martha Vest, for her excellent yoga classes, for giving her time and knowledge to help clearly describe the yoga postures in this book, and for appearing in the photos.

Alexandria Sheeva Ganzel, for swooping down from on high like an angelic eagle to oversee the entire photography project, for making sure that it was finished in record time, and for her skills as a touch-up artist. Her pleasant and gracious demeanor makes her a joy to work with.

My Torah teacher and friend, Gary Shapiro, for making time in his extremely busy life to read my entire manuscript carefully, for his gentle editing skills, and for helping locate sources.

My principal Torah teachers in Jerusalem over the past twenty years: Meir Schweiger, Dov Berkowitz, Shlomo Naeh, Nadine Shenkar, and Marc Kujawski, for their wisdom and inspiration.

Torah scholars and teachers Daniel Matt, Rabbi Yossi Gordon, Rabbi Jonathan Ginsburg, Rabbi Alan Shavit-Lonstein, and Rabbi Moshe Feller, for helping to clarify ideas and find sources.

Iyengar yoga teacher Margie Siegel, for her precision in teaching and for helping me locate sources.

Pam Lauer, for her gentle and beautiful prayers, for trying out all the postures, and for helping to spiritually polish them.

Sara Frailich, for her fresh perspective on the postures used in this book.

All my Torah Yoga students, for sharing my excitement about Torah Yoga and enthusiastically joining me on this new path.

Chris Grey, for his skillful photography; and Sue Grey, for her natural-looking makeup artistry.

Richard Kelly, for his time and willingness to appear in fine form in the photos.

Judith Margolis, for helping me start organizing and writing.

Rolinda Schonwald, for encouraging me and helping me to write before I was ready to write.

All my friends, for cheering me on from all over the world; and in particular, Rena Cohen, for knowing me so well, making me laugh so hard, and loving me so unconditionally; Karin Raveh for her Hebrew expertise; Laura Tota, for her intuitive timing in making the hidden, essential connection that set this book in motion; Revital Gross (Teetan) for loving my daughter and taking care of her the way she does.

My whole family: my loving mother, the world's greatest, tireless listener, for sharing her beautiful home with me and my family, and for her many trips to the grocery store to ensure that we all had something to eat; my daughter, Kalya Tiferet, beautiful, loving and exuberant, for keeping me balanced and for appearing on the cover and in a few photos; Jonathan's daughter, Ruti, in Jerusalem, for her patience and courage while we are so far away from her; my sister Cathy for her excitement about this book; my sister Laura for her appreciation and helpful editing comments; my brother Leon for his belief in me and my work and his legal advice; my brother Ricky for his wholehearted support, even if yoga really isn't his thing; all my loving sisters- and brothers-in-law, nephews, and nieces, for making our family what it is.

My most kind-hearted father, whose memory is a blessing, whose generous and loving spirit has graced so much and so many. He always told me he would help me with Torah Yoga. I am sure he has overseen this entire book.

My grandparents and all my ancestors, for giving me the gift of Judaism.

God, for blessing me with boundless inspiration, enthusiasm, and energy for this work, and in so many other ways.

This book is dedicated to my giant-hearted parents:

Coleman (of blessed memory) and Shirley Bloomfield.

To my father, whose unending faith in me gives me wings for flying.

To my mother, whose unwavering care gives me a home for resting.

# Introduction

*T*ORAH YOGA IS BOTH a Torah book and a yoga book, presenting classic yoga instruction in the light of traditional and mystical Jewish wisdom.

What makes it a unique Torah book is that it actively engages body and breath in the study of Jewish wisdom. It offers guided meditations based on Jewish spiritual concepts. It teaches a wide range of fundamental yoga postures that are suitable for both beginning and advanced students.

What makes it a unique yoga book is its presentation of traditional Jewish study. This includes teaching and quoting directly from Jewish texts and exploring their relationship with yoga. It involves analysis of the original Hebrew letters, words, and phrases, without requiring of the reader any prior familiarity with Hebrew or Torah study.

Torah Yoga is a way to discover and experience yourself through the study of Jewish wisdom, meditation, and yoga.

In the worlds of both Torah and yoga, we are sailing in previously uncharted waters. This book, *Torah Yoga,* is for all those who yearn to explore the open seas.

## Voyage to Torah Yoga

My own voyage to Torah Yoga began when I was a little girl in love with the Hebrew language. Before I knew how to read the Hebrew letters, they looked like fire to me—made of turning, moving, flickering shapes. When we went to synagogue, I gazed with rapt attention at the dancing flames of the Hebrew letters in the prayer book. Some letters rose high, and some cast shadows downward. Some letters looked like sparks, and some looked like full flames. They radiated warmth and depth. They seemed to fly off the pages of the prayer book right into my soul, igniting it with whispered promises of stories, secrets, and meaning. Even though

I grew up in St. Paul, Minnesota, far away both in time and space from the traditional great centers of Jewish learning, the mystic power of Hebrew was clear to me.

## Black Fire, White Fire

My passion for Hebrew eventually took me straight to the heart of the flames, the Torah itself, which is written in Hebrew. When I first became interested in studying the Torah, the image I had was of big, old books, filled with lots of tiny words. I asked a friend, Gary Shapiro, who had already found great meaning in these tiny words, if he thought I would find spiritual meaning in Torah study. He answered very simply, "Yes."

Not long after asking Gary this question, I enrolled in a yearlong Torah study program at Pardes, an institute of Jewish study in Jerusalem based on the yeshiva, or traditional house of study. As a child, I had seen the fire in the Hebrew letters. As an adult at Pardes, I learned that the Torah itself is described as fire. "The Torah is black fire written on the back of white fire."[1] One way to understand this is that the black fire is the written words of the Torah. The white fire is the expansive silent wisdom between the words.

To my great surprise, and my family's, my one year of study at Pardes turned into five, during which I warmed my mind, heart, and soul by the fire of Torah's radiant wisdom. Gary and I often laughed over my original question. Nevertheless, I began to sense that something was missing.

About this time, I had a dream in which I saw three African women in traditional dress dancing. In my dream, I knew that these women were praying. They were praying with their whole bodies. When I awoke, I knew that I needed to pray and to learn with my whole body as well as with my mind, heart, and soul. First I began to dance, and then I turned to yoga.

## First Impressions of Yoga

I first saw yoga when I was twelve years old. Yoga was just appearing on the horizon in the United States, and my older sister, Laura, took a class. She used to practice her postures in our living room. I loved watching her. She looked calm and beautiful. There was an ethereal and mysterious look about her, something soft in the expression on her face and in her eyes.

Watching my sister—poised, balanced, and quiet in her postures—I sensed that yoga was a way to understand something deeper about life. I felt that what she was doing had something to do with knowing God. I knew that someday I would do yoga.

It was many years before I saw yoga again. My friend Myriam Klotz was in my living room practicing yoga. Once again, I was drawn to the mysterious, soft beauty of a person in a yoga posture. I sensed energy, like a gentle, good light, radiating from her. I wanted to experience for myself what these beautiful postures felt like. At that point, I knew the time for me to do yoga had arrived. I went to my first class soon after. Before long, I was practicing yoga every day, as I still do.

## Seeing Yoga with Torah-Centered Eyes

My deep immersion in Judaism gave me a different lens through which to see and experience yoga. Every time I heard a yoga teacher speak about some of the principles of yoga, my yiddishe kop (Jewish head) immediately located where this teaching was in Torah texts. One time, I shared this awareness with an Indian yoga teacher. "Everything you are saying is in Torah," I exclaimed, rather awestruck by the connections. "Of course it is," he replied.

Although yoga is often linked with Vedic, Hindu, Buddhist, and even New Age spirituality and philosophy, B.K.S. Iyengar, one of the foremost yoga masters of our time, says, "Yoga was given for the human race, not for the Hindus."[2] His daughter, Geeta S. Iyengar, says, "Yoga is not Hinduism, or any other ism. It is something eternal."[3] In other words, although yoga is certainly spiritual, it is not tied to any one particular religion.

Students of diverse religious backgrounds flock to India to learn yoga. The great teachers there often tell them that yoga can enhance their connection to their own religion, their own roots.

## Experiencing Torah with Yoga-Centered Body

With yoga, I discovered that the wisdom of Torah was also inside me. I experienced Torah teachings as a reality that I could know and feel within myself, within my body. Because Torah was within me, practicing yoga was a new way to study Torah. Every yoga posture was a gateway to greater Torah consciousness.

The more yoga I practiced, the more Torah I understood at a deeper level, a level that included my body as well as my mind, heart, and soul. I felt that the quiet inner expanse I experienced in yoga was the white fire of the Torah scroll. From the white fire, the black letters of the Torah became increasingly clearer to me.

## Knowing Worlds in Yourself

The twelfth-century Torah commentator from Spain, Ibn Ezra, realized the importance of the body on the spiritual path of wisdom long before it dawned on me: "The one who knows the secret of his soul and the characteristics of his body can know things of the upper world, because the human being is a little world."[4] With Torah Yoga, you study the secrets of your soul and the characteristics of your body. Through the study and experience of your own personal "little world," you can know things of the "upper world."

While sitting by a gigantic sunflower, I envisioned teaching Torah and yoga together, which I have been doing ever since. This book presents Torah Yoga inspirations from the past twelve years of teaching.

## Torah Yoga for You

Although some aspects of Torah, especially the laws and customs, are particular to the Jewish people, much of the wisdom of Torah is universal. Torah itself teaches that the light of Torah, its wisdom, is for all nations. The Torah themes for this book are all universally relevant.

I have taught Jews, Christians, and people of other religions, with varying levels of commitment to their faith, as well as people with little or no connection to any formal religion. Men and women of all ages participate in Torah Yoga classes. I have taught those blessed with good health as well as those who are struggling with illness.

People enjoy Torah Yoga for many reasons. Those of different religions, as well as those who have no connection to any formal religion, are inspired by the universal Jewish teachings. Some students are grateful to find a yoga class that draws from the Judeo-Christian heritage rather than Hindu, Buddhist, or other sources. Some students deeply involved in yoga, but not Judaism, are surprised and pleased to find inspiration and meaning in Jewish wisdom through Torah Yoga. Some students deeply involved with Jewish study and practice are moved, even to tears, when they discover that their own bodies are expressions of Torah wisdom. Many students, estranged from their bodies, are surprised and pleased to discover that they *have* bodies, and that they can gain strength, flexibility, wisdom, and a sense of well-being by connecting to them.

## What Happens in Torah Yoga?

Torah Yoga classes usually consist of several minutes of warm-up postures, a few minutes of meditation on a Torah subject, a question-and-answer study session based on Jewish texts, and then a full yoga session. Doing yoga takes up about three-quarters of the class time.

In this book, I teach seven central Jewish spiritual concepts: hidden light, constant renewal, leaving Egypt, essential self, body prayer and alignment, daily crowns that adorn the letters in the written Torah scroll. Many teachings can only be understood with reference to the Hebrew. For this reason, I use Hebrew in many of the Torah teachings in this book.

## God's Name—YHVH

Torah contains many names for God. God's name written with the Hebrew letters *yud, heh, vav,* and *heh* is known as the ineffable (unutterable) name. In English, it is sometimes transliterated as YHVH. Because this name cannot be said, when studying or reading a text that includes it, many people simply say *hashém* (the name). During formal prayer or when reading from the Torah, it is customary to say *adonái* (Lord) or *elohím* (God).

In Jewish thought, names are considered an expression of the essence of something or someone. God's essence, of course, is ineffable. In this book, I have chosen to acknowledge the ineffable nature of God and to hint at God's mystery and power by using YHVH whenever this name of God appears in this book.

According to traditional Jewish law (Halacha), when the ineffable name of God is written down, it must be treated with respect. For this reason, when a Torah scroll or prayer book becomes damaged or unusable, it should not be thrown away; it must be placed in a *geníza* (archive)—in essence, a special grave for holy texts. This book actually contains one occurrence of *yud, heh, vav,* and *heh* written in Hebrew. However, since the letters are written on top of one another (to make an illustration) and not horizontally (as a word), the law does not apply.

## Torah in the Present Tense

During their journey in the desert, God *gave* Moses and the Children of Israel the Torah at Mount Sinai. We see, however, that in daily Jewish prayers, we bless God, who *gives* the Torah. This indicates that the revelation of Torah began at Sinai, but it did not end there. God is continually giving Torah. God is giving Torah this very moment. For this reason, I have translated many Torah quotes in this book into present tense. For example: "On the first day, God creates light," instead of "On the first day, God created light" (Genesis 1:1–4).

This follows the Jewish mystics' teaching that what sustains the world is the continual utterance of God. God did not say "Let there be light" just one finite time. God, who transcends time and space, is always saying, "Let there be light." Likewise, God did not give the Torah just at one point in time and space. God gives the Torah in every time, in every place, to anyone who is willing to receive it. The mystics imagine God teaching and speaking Torah continually; without God's continual divine utterance, the world would cease to exist.[11]

There is another unconventional usage of present tense in this book. During traditional Jewish study, the ancient sages are usually cited as speaking in the present tense—even if they died centuries ago. For example: one would say, "Rabbi Akiva says, . . ." rather than "Rabbi Akiva said. . . ." This brings our teachers right into the room with us. As we enter into conversation with ancient sages from many places, they live here and now in our Torah study.

Torah is not God's fossilized word preserved in ancient books. It is a participatory tale of communication, interaction, and love between God and creation. The revelation of Torah is the ongoing story of your life and mine.

## Torah Yoga and the Whispers of Existence

> All existence whispers to me a secret:
> I have life to offer—take it, take it . . .
> Arise, and live, and sing to beauty and to life . . .
> Draw delight unending from the dew of heaven.
>
> —RAV KOOK

In our time, the gentle sounds of life have too often been drowned under a cacophony of pain and destruction. Thank God, there are many ways to rise up like the phoenix from the ashes and to hear again the whispered symphony of life-affirming secrets. There are many ways to sing the song of life.

Torah is a way. Torah is called the Tree of Life. Her wise branches rustle and whisper secrets full of life to all who listen.

Yoga is also a way. With yoga, you can hear your own breath and body whispering to you: I have life to offer—take it, take it.

With these ancient and ever renewing whisperers of life, Torah and yoga, you can rise up with a joyful and renewed body-mind-heart-soul. This book, *Torah Yoga,* is for all those who want to draw delight from the dance of life.

# Using This Book

FOR ME, TORAH STUDY and yoga practice are part of a way of life that is filled with searching for and finding meaning, purpose, and joy. The way is at least as important as any particular benefit or goal. Therefore, this book is not intended simply as a how-to tool for achieving a particular result such as more knowledge, spirituality, strength, or flexibility.

This book is also not meant to take the place of live Torah or yoga instruction. I am continually studying both Torah and yoga from many texts and with many different teachers.

Actually, there are many different satisfying and beneficial ways to use and read this book, depending on the reader. Whatever way serves your own particular interests and needs is the best way for you.

Here are a few possible approaches:

- Start with and read only whatever subjects interest you most right now. It is not necessary to read the chapters in any particular order.

- Open the book and read at random. Perhaps the particular page you open to will turn out not to be so random after all.

- Read it cover to cover. Study and practice one chapter each day of the week, ending with Chapter Seven, which is about Shabbat (Friday night to Saturday night), and remembering to rest.

However you approach the book, you can read and use it over and over, continually gaining benefits and insights from both the yoga practice and the text study.

## Keys to Hebrew Transliteration and Pronunciation

This book requires no familiarity with Hebrew. Everything you need to know is explained as you read along. For those interested, here are the keys to its transliteration and pronunciation.

Hebrew has its own alphabet just as, for example, Greek does. To enable everyone to read the Hebrew words or phrases in this book, they are transliterated using English letters and shown in ***bold italics***. Immediately after the first instance of a transliterated Hebrew word or phrase, you usually find its English translation in parentheses. Examples: ***olám*** (world) and ***katán*** (little). Note that Hebrew word order often differs from English word order. For example, in Hebrew, adjectives usually come after nouns. As a result, phrase translations often do not preserve the original Hebrew word order. Example: ***olám katán*** (little world).

Although English letters are used for the Hebrew words in this book, the resulting words are not pronounced like English words. Here is the pronunciation guide:

- All single-letter vowels should be pronounced as in Italian: *a* as in *mama*, *e* as in *wet*, *i* as in *pique*, *o* as in *toe*, and *u* as in *duke*.

- The only double letter vowels used are *ei* or *ey*, as in *sleigh* or *hey*, and *ai* or *ay*, as in *aisle* or *aye*.

- An apostrophe between two consonants represents the vowel sound *uh*— as in *up*.

- An apostrophe between two vowels represents a slight beat—as in the second *o* of *cooperate*.

- There is only one accented syllable per word; an accent mark over the accented vowel shows where it is.

- The letter combination *ch* always sounds as in *Bach*, never as it does in *cheese*.

- All other consonantal letters used *(b, d, f, g, h, k, l, m, n, p, r, s, t, v, y, z)* are pronounced just as they are in English.

Although many transliterated Hebrew words appear in this book, there are only a few transliterated Sanskrit words. English terms are used for all yoga postures. Although the Sanskrit language has its own depth, beauty, and wisdom, Sanskrit is simply beyond the scope and purpose of this book.

## Resources

At the end of the book, you will find the following resources for further study.

Reading the meditations and postures in this book and simultaneously trying to do them is not recommended. One alternative is to record yourself or someone else reading the text and then to do the yoga by listening to the recording. Another is to have one person read the instructions aloud while you do them; then switch roles. This way you can gain mastery of the postures by studying them from the text, observing another person doing them, and practicing them yourself. This method resembles the traditional Jewish method of learning with a *chevrúta* (friend).

## More About Breath

Yoga has many techniques for conscious breathing or control of breath. The most important instruction for conscious breathing in this book is simple—remember to breathe!

It is natural to stop breathing when you feel tension or distress, but holding your breath will only increase the tension you feel. Yoga can teach you to move beyond your natural tendency. It can teach you to become conscious of your breath and to learn to notice when you are holding it. Remember to breathe, especially when you feel tension; in fact, breathe right into the places that feel tense. Breathe in and out through your nose. Breathe naturally and steadily. Relax your breath; relax yourself.

## How Long to Hold a Posture

Rather than suggesting an amount of time to hold each posture, I have suggested a certain number of breaths. This will help keep your focus inward and on your breath as you deepen into your postures, rather than outward on a clock.

Above all, follow your own intuition in deciding how long to hold a posture. Trust yourself. You know what is best for you.

## Individualizing Your Practice

In general, yoga is beneficial for everyone. However, all postures are not always appropriate. Some days, challenging postures are just what you want. Other days, restorative postures are more fitting. Tune your practice to your own changing needs and rhythms.

As a further refinement, adjust each posture to suit you. My instructions are pointing you in a particular direction. However, yoga is not about achieving a particular form in a posture. You are doing yoga when you listen well to your body. Trust your intuition as you navigate your way through the postures.

CHAPTER

# The Hidden Light

# האור הגנוז

ON THE FIRST DAY OF CREATION, according to the book of Genesis, God creates light. On the fourth day of creation, God creates the sun, moon, and stars. If this light of the first day of creation is not sunlight, moonlight, or starlight, what is it? Where is it? Does it have any meaning for us now?

Jewish mystics teach that the first light is connected to God's essence. Because the first light is so powerful, God hides it. The mystics call it *haór haganúz* (the hidden light). However, the hidden light can be found. It can be found everywhere. Most importantly, it can be found in you.

With the practice of yoga, you can look for, find, and reveal to the world the power and beauty of the mysterious hidden light within you.

## ⌒ Your Own Body of Wisdom

Take a moment to play hide and seek with yourself. You are the seeker. Find out some things about yourself: Can you recall a time when you felt powerful and radiant? Have you ever felt too small to receive someone's generosity or love? What is your most hidden mystery? Turn to your own wisdom sources for the answers to these questions. Consider your own body as a source of wisdom. How well do you know it? Your own breath is a mystery. How familiar are you with it?

**Torah Yoga for the Hidden Light**

According to the Ari, a sixteenth-century mystic in Sefad, Israel, God desires to shower the world with the abundant goodness of the hidden light. In order to give this light, God "needs" a vessel capable of receiving it.[1] In this world-view, your task is to build yourself into a vessel of receptivity.

Although babies and children are usually soft bundles of receptivity, it is not always easy or simple to receive loving-kindness and goodness as we grow older. Many things happen that tend to harden us and close us down. Great gifts, even small gifts, can be overwhelming. However, receptivity is something you can practice and relearn. Yoga is training in receptivity. As well as making you strong, yoga can transform you into a soft, open, receptive vessel for the hidden light.

## Vessel Making

In Jewish High Holiday liturgy, God is described as a potter who fashions his creations. Pottery is a very old craft for vessel making. Yoga is also a craft for vessel making. With yoga, you become a pottery partner with God and participate in making the vessel of yourself.

In ordinary pottery, you work with clay. What do you work with in the pottery of yoga? Your body, of course, can be likened to clay that you stretch and mold. However, as you work with your body, you realize that your body is not separate from your mind, heart, and soul. Your breath helps to soften and release your body. Your thoughts and emotions contribute to the texture and pliability of your body. For example, if you say to yourself, "I am not flexible," your body will probably believe you and not move so easily. If, on the other hand, you say to yourself, "I am open and yielding," your body may very well open and yield. If you are afraid, your body tightens up. If you feel safe, your body relaxes. Yoga is a physical, mental, emotional, and spiritual experience all at once. Your body-mind-heart-soul is the raw material on the yoga pottery wheel.

With yoga, you are involved in fashioning your own vessel: yourself. When you work often with the clay of your whole self, you become both a soft and a strong vessel—a vessel capable of receiving and revealing to the world the mysterious hidden light of the first day of creation.

## Hidden Light Within You

Though you may not be aware of it, you are already a vessel containing hidden light. Jewish tradition teaches that each human being is an ***olám katán*** (little world). The Malbim, a nineteenth-century Torah commentator in Poland, says: "the whole of reality is organized and arranged like the structure of a human being, because the human being is a *little world* that includes within itself all the powers that are found in all the worlds."[2] In another teaching, the Malbim says: "Each person is a metaphor, image, and imitation of the whole big world."[3]

Because you are a little world, within you are all the powers that are found in all the worlds—within you is the hidden light of the first day of creation. Yoga is a way to discover the hidden light within you.

## Mystery of the Hidden Light

Jewish mystics have a lot to say about the hidden light. It is abundant love. It is divine consciousness. It is a mystery connected to God's seemingly paradoxical presence and hiddenness in the world and in our lives. This mystery is within you. Yoga begins with a stretch of your spine and a deep breath and continues inward to the hidden and not completely knowable mystery of God within you. In the Torah, Job (19:26) speaks of the experience of seeing God with his body: "In my flesh I see God." Rav Kook, first chief rabbi of Israel and the great mystic poet and sage of the last century, writes about his own intimate experience of the light: "My secret is for me—and my secret is my light—and my light is with me—the treasure of my life."[4] Let Torah and yoga guide you to the hidden treasure within you.

 ## Torah Study for the Hidden Light

What is the light of the first day of creation? In the Talmud, Rabbi Eliezer teaches: "In the light that the Holy One, Blessed be He, created on the first day of creation, a person can see from one end of the world to the other."[5] The original Hebrew text also means that one can see from the start of creation to its end. In other words, the first light illuminates all space and time. It enables absolute seeing, or God consciousness.

According to the primary text of Jewish mysticism, the *Zohar*, the first light is *chésed* (loving-kindness).[6] God desires to pour this loving-kindness into the world in great abundance. The mystics teach that the ability of the giver to give is in direct correlation to the ability of the receiver to receive. God wants people to learn to be receptive.[7] God wants vessels that are prepared and open to hold divine love.

The vessel is a central image in Jewish mysticism. The world and human beings are seen as vessels that need to prepare themselves to receive love. The more the vessel can contain, the more love is poured in.

We can also understand the first light as God's clothing. The psalmist writes: "He wraps Himself in light as a garment" (Psalms 104:2). In the Midrash, the rabbis say: ". . . the Holy One, Blessed be He, wraps Himself in a white garment and shines the radiant light of His glory from one end of the world to the other."[8]

The first four letters of the Hebrew alphabet also hint at this story of God coming into the world clothed. The first letter, *aleph*, symbolizes oneness, unity, mystery, and, in fact, God. Following *aleph*, we have the letters *bet, gimel,* and *dalet*, which together spell *bégged* (clothing). So *aleph, bet, gimel,* and *dalet*, can be read as *aleph bégged* (God clothed).

The first light, then, can be seen as God's garment radiating the light of divine consciousness and love into the world.

## Mystical Dilemma of God's Presence

Why does God need a garment of light in order to come into the world? Why doesn't God come in directly? This question touches on a central dilemma of Jewish mysticism. The mystics teach that God is *ein sof* (without end). The mystical dilemma is this: How can infinite God interact with finite creation without overwhelming it? If God were fully in the world, there would be no room for creation.[9] One answer to this dilemma is the first light. It is God's way of interacting and communicating with finite creation.

The mystics understand that even the first light, if fully revealed, would be too powerful for the unprepared world.[10] Our world is not strong enough to hold God's garment of light without preparation. If the first light poured in directly, it would break our unprepared world as if it were a lightbulb given too much power for its capacity. In the Talmud, the rabbis also teach that God saw potential misuse of this first great light.[11] Therefore, God hides the first light. The psalmist writes: "How great is the goodness that you have hidden for those who revere you" (Psalms 31:20). The *Zohar* says this hidden goodness is the first light.[12]

The concept of the hidden light is hinted at in the Hebrew word *olám* (world). This word is built from the three-letter root *áyin, lámed, mem.* The root itself means "hidden" or "concealed." Why does the Hebrew word for *world* allude to concealment? What is truly hidden in our world? The hidden light, of course— all the aspects of God that are contained in the powerful, illuminating, and potentially shattering first light.

## Where Is the Hidden Light?

The great first light is in hiding. Where is it? How can we find it and let it shine forth from its hiding place? There are many answers to these questions.

The psalmist says, "And the light is sown for the righteous" (Psalms 97:11). Referring to the first light, the Talmud also teaches: "And God hid it for the righteous."[13] We learn from tradition that Moses is one righteous man who not only found the hidden light but also revealed it to others. Does all this mean that the hidden light is only for a select few? How many people can be righteous like Moses?

Maimonides, the great codifier and philosopher from twelfth-century Spain, teaches: "Every person is fit to be righteous like Moses."[14] The hidden light, therefore, is sown potentially for every person.

The Baal Shem Tov, the eighteenth-century Eastern European founder of the Hasidic movement, says that the first light is hidden in the Torah. "Where did the Blessed Holy One hide it (the first light)? He hid it in the Torah."[15] The book of Proverbs teaches, "Torah is light" (6:23). To study Torah and to follow its teachings is a way to find and reveal the hidden light.

## Moses and the Hidden Light

The Torah, which some say *is* the first light, also tells of the revealing of the first light in the story of Moses. Moses brings the children of Israel out of the darkness of Egyptian slavery so that they can receive the light of the Torah at Mount Sinai.

One of the first connections between Moses and the first light comes at his birth: "And the woman got pregnant, and she gave birth to a son, and she saw that he was good, and she hid him for three months" (Exodus 2:2). Rashi, the eleventh-century Torah commentator in France, says, "When he was born the whole house filled up with light."[16] Why does Rashi, known for explaining the plain meaning of the text, bring in the notion of light in connection with Moses' birth? The text does not mention light directly. What is he basing his comment on?

Rashi hears an echo reverberating through the text from the first day of creation. When Moses is born, the text says, "and she saw that he was good" (Exodus 2:2). When God creates light, the text says: "And God saw that the light was good" (Genesis 1:4). From this linguistic echo, Rashi connects the word *good* with light—and not just any light—the first light, the light of God. Moses' birth heralds the revealing of the first light into the world.

Just as the first light has to be concealed until there is a vessel to contain it, Moses has to be concealed after his birth: "and she hid him for three months" (Exodus 2:2). Again, the light was too powerful for the unprepared world to contain all at once. The light that Moses radiated when he was born was a foreshadowing of his life's purpose. Moses grew to become a vessel not only strong enough to receive Torah, the first light, but also strong enough to reveal it to the world.

### Receive and Reveal the Hidden Light

Torah *is* the first light and a guide to finding the first light. Sfat Emet, the nineteenth-century Hasidic Rebbe of Gur, Poland, teaches, "Human beings are created to give light in this world."[17] Everyone can fill the house with light as Moses did. With the teachings of Torah, one can learn how to become a vessel strong enough to receive and reveal the first light.

May we all discover our own path to the first light and together develop the strength to fill the whole world with it.

## Yoga Practice for the Hidden Light

Move now to the practice of yoga, with the intention of making yourself a vessel for receiving and revealing more of the hidden light.

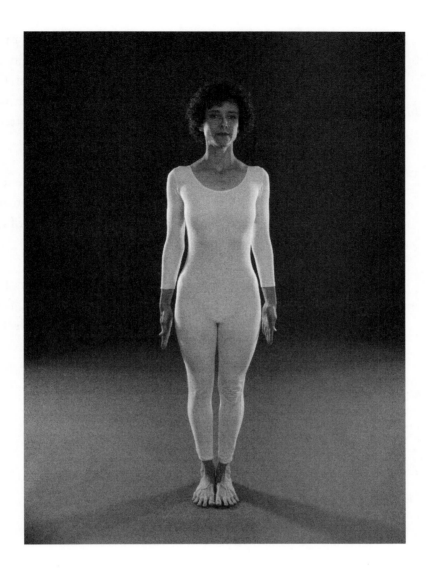

# Mountain Posture

Stand with the inner edges of your feet together. Broaden and lengthen the soles of your feet, and stretch and spread your toes. Lift the inner arches of your feet up. Distribute your weight evenly over the heels and balls of your feet. Press your heels into the floor, and stretch your legs up vertically. Pull the front of your thighs up, lifting your kneecaps.

Move your tailbone down and in. Move your hips back over your heels. Bring equal weight to both feet. Take a few breaths to feel the connection you are making with the earth.

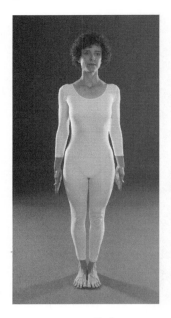

**Photo 2.1**

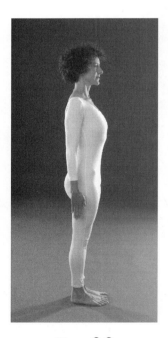

**Photo 2.2**

Roll your shoulders back, and actively stretch your arms down by your sides all the way through your fingertips, palms facing in. Move your shoulder blades in toward your chest, and lift your chest. On an inhalation, stretch your spine upward, lengthening the sides of your waist. Press your back ribs in, and breathe into your expanding chest. Soften your belly (Photo 2.1).

Relax your forehead, soften your eyes, and feel the energy within you. Breathe evenly into your whole body for three to five breaths as you root, lengthen, and expand. Imagine yourself as a vessel full of light. Be receptive to your own inner light (Photo 2.2).

Now release the actions of the posture and take a moment to notice and absorb the benefits. Be attentive to changes inside. Yoga is training in attentiveness. Whatever is happening, whether it be subtle or strong, notice it and receive it.

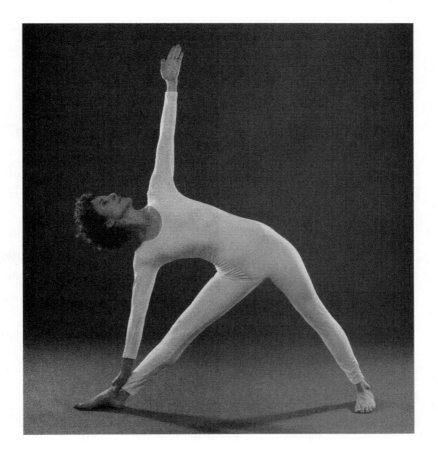

# Triangle Posture

Bring your feet together and stand in Mountain Posture (see this chapter, Photos 2.1–2.2). Gather your attention inward.

Jump or step your feet four to four and a half feet apart. At the same time, extend your arms out sideways, parallel to the floor, palms facing down. Turn your toes in slightly, heels out, so that the outer edges of your feet are parallel to each other (Photo 3.1).

Turn your left foot twenty degrees to the right. Turn your right leg and foot ninety degrees to the right. Line up your right heel with the arch of your left foot.

Press your feet firmly into the floor, and straighten both legs. Pull the fronts of your thighs up, lifting your

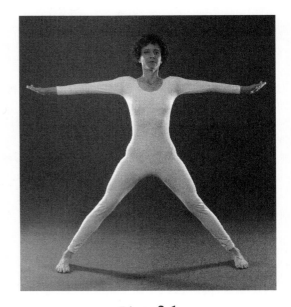

**Photo 3.1**

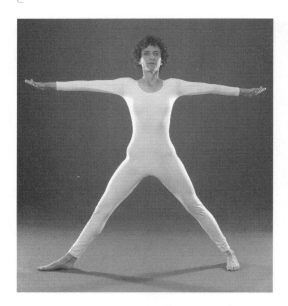

**Photo 3.2**

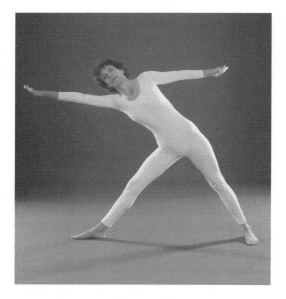

**Photo 3.3**

kneecaps. Rotate the fronts of your thighs away from each other. The front of your right thigh and knee should face to the right. The front of your left thigh and knee should face forward.

Move your tailbone in and down. Check that the front of your torso and pelvis face forward and that your pelvis is level. On an inhalation, lift your waist up away from your pelvis and extend the sides of your torso up evenly.

Stretch your arms out from the middle of your chest to your fingertips. Broaden and lift your chest as your arms lengthen out to your sides (Photo 3.2).

Inhale and lengthen your spine even more. Exhale and extend your torso out over the line of your right leg (Photo 3.3).

Continuing to lengthen the right side of your torso, bring your right hand down to your calf or ankle or to a block or the floor behind your right ankle. Keep your left thigh back and tuck your right buttocks under. Stretch your left arm up directly over your left shoulder, palm facing forward. Face forward. Breathe evenly, and open up from the inside out.

Press the outer edge of your left foot into the floor, and straighten and firm your left leg. Press the inner edge of your right foot into the floor, and straighten and firm your right leg. Continually tuck your right buttocks under.

On an inhalation, stretch your spine from your tailbone to the crown of your head, lengthening your trunk out to the right. Turn the right side of your torso forward and the left side of your torso back. Then turn your head and gaze up at your left hand (Photo 3.4). Relax your face and your eyes.

Be involved in the posture for three to five breaths. Rather than letting the actions of the posture fade away over time, make them stronger the longer you hold the posture. Straighten and firm your legs. Breathe softness into your lengthening, turning spine. Affirm to yourself: "I am strong and open."

To release, press your feet firmly into the floor, stretch your left arm up toward the ceiling, and on an inhalation come up to standing. Release your arms down to your sides. Turn your feet to face forward. Walk them in a little, and then either jump or walk them back together. Soften inside and notice how you feel. Be open to receive the gifts this posture offers you.

Repeat this posture on the other side.

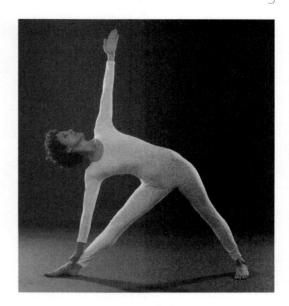

**Photo 3.4**

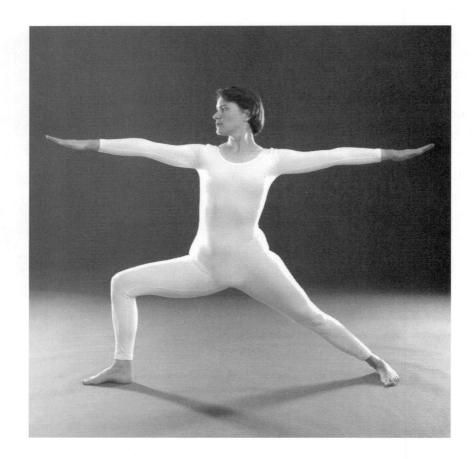

# Warrior Two Posture

Bring your feet together and stand in Mountain Posture (see this chapter, Photos 2.1–2.2). Take a few breaths to turn your attention to your whole body.

Jump or step your feet four and a half to five feet apart. Turn your toes in, heels out, so that the outer edges of your feet run parallel to each other.

Place your hands on your hips. Turn your left foot twenty degrees to the right and your right leg and foot ninety degrees to the right. Press both feet firmly into the floor. Pull the front of your thighs up, and lift your kneecaps. Straighten both legs, and rotate the fronts of your thighs away from each other.

Extend your arms out to your sides with your palms facing the floor. Stretch from the center of your chest out to your fingertips, and keep your shoulders down and away from your ears (Photo 4.1). Check that your torso is facing forward and that your pelvis is level.

On an inhalation, lengthen your spine, creating a longer waist. On an exhalation, bend your right knee to a ninety-degree angle, moving your knee into a position directly above your right ankle. Tuck your right buttock under, and stretch your inner right thigh from your groin to your knee.

Press into the outer edge of your left foot, and stretch your left leg upward. Keep rotating the fronts of your thighs away from each other.

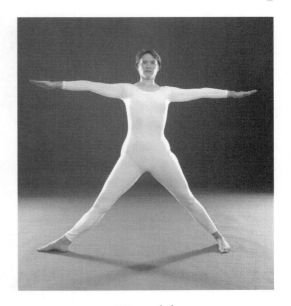

**Photo 4.1**

While maintaining the ninety-degree bend of your right knee, inhale and extend your spine up. Draw your shoulder blades into your back, and lift and expand your chest. Check that the front of your torso is facing forward and that your pelvis is level.

Stretch your left arm to the left as you turn your head to the right, and gaze out beyond your right fingertips (Photo 4.2). Relax your forehead, eyes, and jaw. Quiet your thinking mind. Become absorbed in the sensations of this posture.

Continually energize the actions of this posture for three to five breaths, breathing steadily and evenly. Feel your strength, your radiant energy. Be a warrior for light.

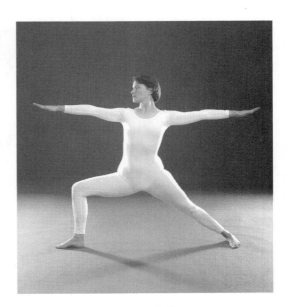

**Photo 4.2**

To release, press your left foot into the floor, inhale, and straighten your right leg to come up to standing. Turn your feet to face forward. Walk your feet in a bit, and then jump or walk your feet back together. Take a moment to absorb the benefits of the posture.

Repeat on the second side.

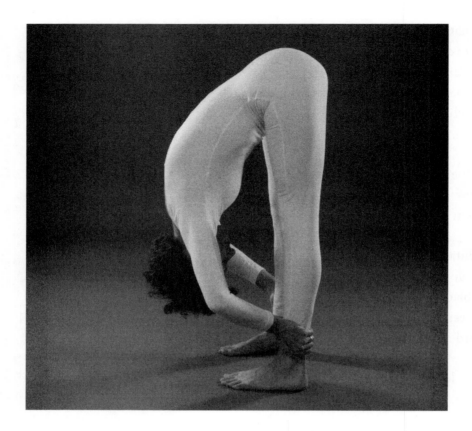

# Standing Forward Bend

### Stage One

Bring your feet together and stand in Mountain Posture (see this chapter, Photos 2.1–2.2). Take a few breaths to center your attention. Press your heels into the floor, and stretch your legs and spine upward.

Step your feet hip-width apart. Turn your toes in slightly, heels out, so that the outer edges of your feet run parallel to each other. Lengthen and broaden your feet, and spread and stretch your toes. Press your heels firmly into the floor, and pull the front of your thighs up, lifting your kneecaps. Rotate the fronts of your thighs in toward each other.

On an inhalation, raise your arms up over your head, palms facing each other, arms parallel. Inhale again, and lift the front and back sides of your spine upward. Take a few breaths here, coordinating your inhalations with lengthening your spine.

On an exhalation, lengthen the front of your spine, and lead with your chest as you bend forward at your hips, extending your trunk forward and down. Place the tips of your fingers on the floor or on blocks so that your hands are directly below your shoulders. Press the tips of your fingers down, and stretch your arms up away from the floor.

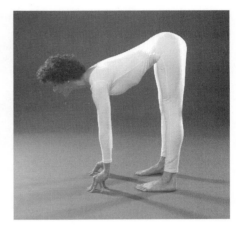

Bring your weight forward so that your hips are aligned directly above your heels. Then press your heels into the floor, and stretch your legs up again. Lift your head and chest.

Inhale and actively stretch your legs up, lifting your kneecaps. Rotate your upper thighs inward, and then press your thighs back as you stretch your spine and chest forward (Photo 5.1).

Breathe evenly, quiet your mind, feel your body getting more involved in the stretch. Breathe into places that feel tight or resistant. This is the concave part of the posture.

**Photo 5.1**

## Stage Two

Hold the backs of your ankles or calves with your hands. Bend your elbows, and lift them out to the sides. On an inhalation, lengthen the front of your spine. On an exhalation, draw your trunk down and in toward your legs. Release your head down, top of your head facing the floor, and relax the back of your neck.

Bring your hips forward over the line of your heels. Actively stretch your legs upward as your spine passively elongates downward (Photo 5.2). Soften your belly. Relax your face, your eyes, and your jaw.

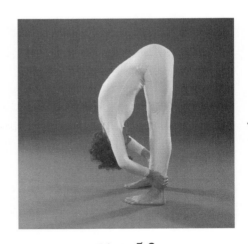

Hold this posture for three to five breaths as you move deeper into your body. Do not strain or force yourself. Patiently and gently, breathe into places that feel resistant or closed. Attend to the secrets of your breath and the characteristics of your body.

To release, first come back to the concave part of this posture. Bring your fingertips to the floor or blocks in front

**Photo 5.2**

of you. Press your feet into the floor and extend your chest and spine forward. Lift your head.

To come up all the way, press your feet into the floor. Place your hands on your hips. On an inhalation, extend your trunk forward, and lead with your chest to lift up to standing. Release your hands down by your sides. Relax, and take a moment to notice the impression this posture makes inside you.

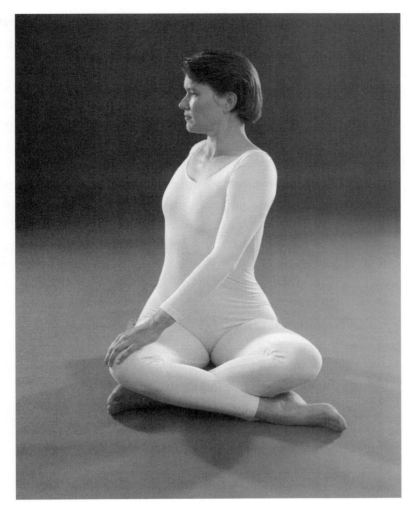

**Photo 6.1**

# Simple Sitting Twist

Sit on a firm blanket with your legs crossed. Have your blanket high enough so that your knees are lower than your hips. Pull the flesh of your buttocks out to the sides and diagonally back. Center yourself evenly on both of your sitz bones. Place your hands down on the floor on either side of your hips, fingers facing forward. Pressing your hands down, use your arms to help extend your spine up. Lift the crown of your head upward.

Roll your shoulders and upper arms back. Press your shoulder blades into your back, inhale, and lift your chest. Soften your belly, the back of your throat, and your eyes.

Place your left hand on top of your right knee. Place your right fingertips down on the floor a few inches behind your left buttock, fingers facing back.

On your inhalations, lengthen your spine upward, creating space between each vertebra. On your exhalations, move more deeply into the twist, turning your whole torso from left to right. Use your hands and arms to assist you in turning.

Keep your shoulders down away from your ears, and lift your elbows out to your sides to make more room for your chest to broaden and expand. Keep your face the same direction that your heart is facing (Photo 6.1). Soften your belly.

Continue to spiral your torso deeper into this posture for five to seven breaths. Inhale and lengthen; exhale and turn. Quiet your mind; relax your face and eyes. As your spine turns, draw your attention inward to the mystery that is you.

To release, return to center slowly with awareness.

Repeat the twist to the second side. Then switch the cross of your legs, and repeat the twist, first to your right and then to your left.

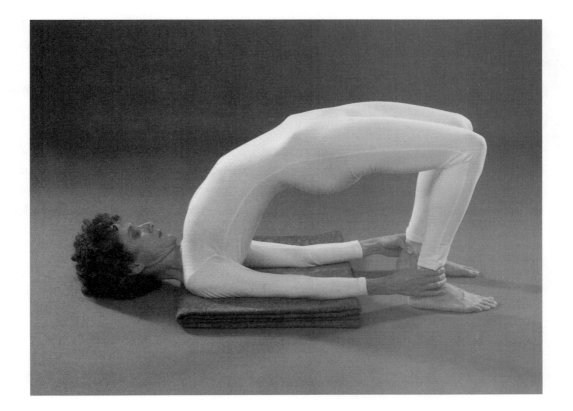

# Bridge Posture

Place a firm folded blanket on the floor. Lie on your back on top of the blanket, bringing the tops of your shoulders to the edge of the blanket, the back of your head on the floor. Bend your knees, and use your hands to bring your heels in close to your buttocks, feet on the floor, hip-width apart. Turn your toes in slightly, heels out, so that the outer edges of your feet are parallel to each other.

With your arms tucked in close to your body, bend your elbows and lift your hands up, fingertips facing the ceiling, palms facing each other. Press the tips of your elbows down into the floor, and lift your chest. Press your shoulder blades in, and move them down toward your waist (Photo 7.1). Relax your face, eyes, and the back of your throat. Turn your attention inward.

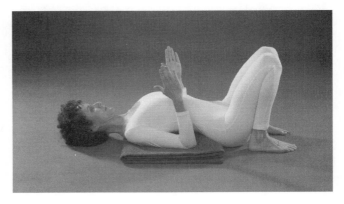

**Photo 7.1**

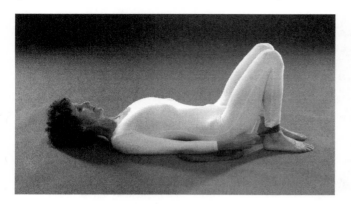

**Photo 7.2**

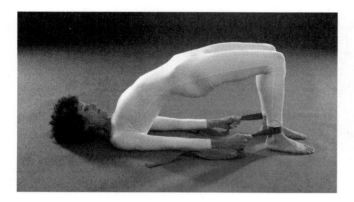

**Photo 7.3**

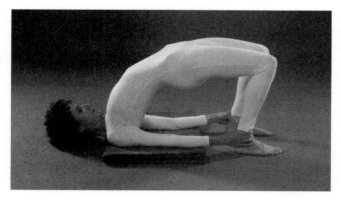

**Photo 7.4**

Stretch your arms toward your feet, and hold your ankles. If you cannot reach them, place a strap around the front of your ankles (Photo 7.2). Hold the strap close to your ankles, and straighten your arms.

On an exhalation, press your shoulders and heels down into the floor, pull on your ankles or the straps, and lift your hips up toward the ceiling. Press your outer arms down. Lift your back ribs up to expand your chest.

Inhale into your expanding chest and roll your shoulders down. Firm your buttocks as you press your tailbone up toward the ceiling. Keep your thighs, knees, and outer edges of your feet parallel to one another, toes slightly turned in. Do not let your knees splay out to the sides.

Lengthen the back of your neck and turn your gaze toward your chest (Photos 7.3–7.4). Relax your throat and eyes. Look within.

Hold yourself up for three to five breaths, breathing evenly. Feel what is happening. Let sensations build. Strengthen your vessel. You are opening windows of awareness throughout your body-mind.

To release, lower your back to the floor; release your legs; relax. Repeat the posture a few times.

When you are finished, rest on your back. Extend your legs onto the floor, and let go of any effort. Soften your eyes, and feel the effects of the posture. Take several minutes to rest, bathing in the abundant light within you.

CHAPTER

# Constant Renewal

## חידוש תמידי

S FAT EMET TEACHES that God creates the world so that every day there is an abundance of new life. He teaches that, in order to appreciate God's daily gift of abundant new life, a person should perceive at the very least one new thing every day. When one perceives something new, one merits feeling something new.[1]

Scientists tell us that the cells in our bodies are continually being renewed. Do you perceive or feel the reality of that renewal? Do you consider yourself new or old? Do you agree with Sfat Emet that "Every day there is renewal,"[2] or do you feel that "There is nothing new under the sun" (Ecclesiastes 1:9)? Whatever your current belief, the practice of yoga can help you to perceive and feel your self-renewal.

People who meditate are fond of quoting the following proverb: "You never step into the same river twice."[3] Every time you step into a river, you are stepping into new waters. Yoga is an immersion in the river of divine renewal flowing through your body. Each time you do a posture, you are stepping into a new river.

### Discovering What's New

What's new with you? Take some time to hear from yourself more than a habitual response to this routinely asked question. What really feels new to you in your life? What feels old? In what areas in your life would you welcome renewal?

Even if you are not currently aware of anything new, yoga can help you to discover renewal that is happening in your life right now.

## Torah Yoga for Constant Renewal

At the end of a traditional Jewish wedding, the groom intentionally steps on a glass cup and breaks it. All the guests call out an exuberant *mazál tov* (good luck). One common explanation for this tradition is that the broken glass is a symbolic remembrance of the destruction of the Temple in Jerusalem.

However, the breaking of the glass cup also symbolizes a break with the old. The bride and groom are breaking the old vessels of their lives so that they can make a new vessel—their new life together. The guests are congratulating the couple as they break with the old and begin the new.

This second explanation actually comes from the Jewish mystical tradition of Kabbalah. Kabbalah teaches that rigid, fixed vessels must break for the sake of renewal. Kabbalah sees the whole world and everything in it as holy vessels containing life. Because the world and everything in it is constantly being renewed—because new life is constantly being created—all rigid, fixed vessels in the world must break so that they can transform into new vessels, vessels ready to hold new life.

Perhaps the Kabbalah's teaching also explains why it is a custom in many Jewish communities to say *mazál tov* whenever anyone breaks a glass—no matter what the occasion!

### Unlock Your Old Habits

Sfat Emet teaches, "The opposite of habit is renewal."[4] Your habits can make you into a rigid, fixed vessel. In a gentle, conscious way, yoga postures can help you to transform your vessel so that it does not break. When you live in habitual ways, you cannot perceive or feel what is new. Habits lock you into perceiving only what you have always perceived. In order to perceive new things, you must change your habitual ways. Yoga is a technique for unlocking your habits in order to perceive the constantly renewing creation both inside and around you.

My friend Shira Rosenschein feels that yoga is like a combination lock that you turn one way to a number, another way to another number, and so on, and then—presto—it opens! Even though the numbers and turns seem random, it works. Likewise, in yoga, you turn part of your body one way, other parts other ways, and so on. Somehow the combination of turns and movements opens the lock and sets you free.

Even without our knowing why it works, every yoga posture is an opportunity to unlock deeply held conscious and unconscious habits. As you unlock the ways you hold your body, habit by habit, you release old perceptions of reality. Without conscious effort, people tend to move through their days in a limited number of habitual body postures. Yoga teaches you to consciously twist, turn, open, and stretch your body in innumerable new ways. Who knows what new life awaits you and your renewed, flowing body!

## Habits of Thought and Emotion

People also tend to have habitual postures of thought and emotion. Thoughts such as "I am not flexible" or "I am not strong" encourage the body to remain in old habits. Fears such as "I am afraid I will hurt myself if I move in this way" are sometimes only emotional habits. Your body may be fixed by a memory of a time when a certain position was not safe or good for you. In the present moment, however, that fixed memory may not be relevant to the possibilities in your body. By changing old messages that you tell yourself, you change your perception of reality.

## Body-Centered Perception

Perception is not located somewhere between your chin and the top of your head. Your eyes are not the sole determiner of how you see. Your whole body is your field of perception. Every cell in your body participates in the way you perceive your reality. If your body is locked in old habits, you see the world out of old-body eyes.

Yoga is a way to perceive and experience renewal every day. In my daily yoga practice, I am continually astounded as I touch the pulse of renewing creation beating in my body. Because I am a part of renewing creation, even if I repeat the same posture day after day, year after year, I always experience something new.

Consider yourself as a vessel containing life. If you hold yourself fixed and rigid, you may, for a while, prevent the new life trying to come in, but eventually you will break. With the practice of yoga, you can continually transform yourself. You can keep yourself open to the constant renewal of life within you.

##  Torah Study for Constant Renewal

"And in His goodness, God is continually renewing creation every day."[5] This affirmation of divine constant renewal is said daily in traditional Jewish prayers. Yet Ecclesiastes 1:9 seems to contradict this: "There is nothing new under the sun." What is the resolution to the apparent contradiction between "God is constantly renewing creation every day" and "There is nothing new under the sun?"

## Perception Is a Key

Rav Kook says: "The perception that dawns on a person—to see the world not as finished, but as in the process of continually becoming, ascending, developing—this [perception] raises him from being 'under the sun' to being 'above the sun'—from the place where there is nothing new, to the place where there is nothing old—where everything takes on new form."[6]

Rav Kook speaks of a "perception that dawns on a person." In Rav Kook's view, whether you live in the place of everything new or nothing new is determined by how you perceive reality. One resolution of this apparent contradiction, then, lies in your perception. When you have the "perception that dawns on a person," everything looks new; without it, nothing looks new.

## Acquire the Perception for Newness

How does one acquire the perception for newness? How does one actually rise to a place above the sun—a place where there is nothing old? The Torah itself teaches us ways to reach the place above the sun. Let us turn to the story of Moses at the burning bush. When Moses turns aside to look at the burning bush, God says to him, "Take your shoes off your feet, the place you are standing on is holy ground" (Exodus 3:5).

The Hebrew word *ná'al* (shoe) is built from the root letters *nun, áyin,* and *lámed.* The verb form of this root means "to lock." The Hebrew word *régel* (foot) is built from the root letters *resh, gímel,* and *lámed.* These root letters are also used for the Hebrew word *hergél* (habit). "Take your shoes off your feet" can also be understood as "Take the locks off your habits." Moses is about to receive his divine mission to go and free the children of Israel from slavery in Egypt. God's first instruction to Moses on this mission is "Take the locks off your habits."

As we learned earlier, Sfat Emet teaches: "The opposite of habit is renewal."[7] God's first instruction to Moses is a key for learning to perceive newness. God tells Moses to unlock his habits so that he can perceive new realities for himself and for the Jewish people. As he learns to unlock his habits, Moses is able to teach the children of Israel to unlock theirs. By taking their shoes off their feet, or unlocking their habits, the Children of Israel move to the world above the sun—a world of constant renewal.

## Watch for the New Moon

When the Jews leave Egypt, God points to the new moon, the start of a new lunar month, and says: "This month is for you" (Exodus 12:2). The Hebrew word *chódesh* (month) is built from the root *chet, dálet, shin.* The root itself means "new." The

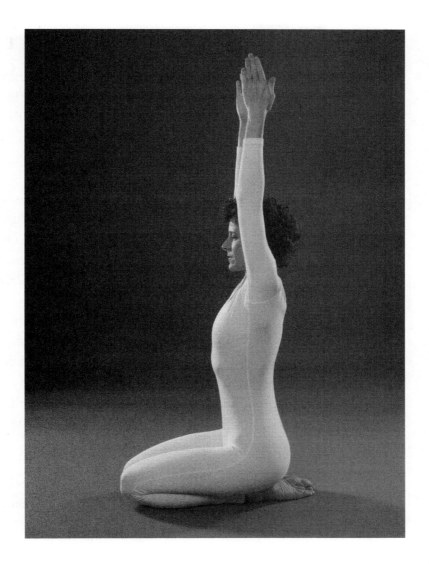

# Seated Mountain Posture

Come onto your hands and knees. Bring your knees and toes together, and sit back on your heels. Inhale and lengthen your spine upward, shoulders over your hips.

If there is too much discomfort or strain on the tops of your feet or ankles, place a blanket or two underneath your shins, with the tops of your feet hanging over the back edge of the blanket.

If your buttocks do not reach your heels, or if there is too much discomfort or strain on your knees, place a blanket between your thighs and calves, wedged up to the inner crease of your knees (see Photo 8.3 for blanket placement).

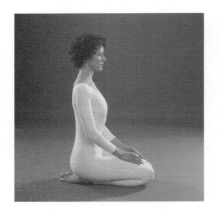

**Photo 8.1**

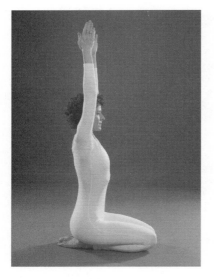

**Photo 8.2**

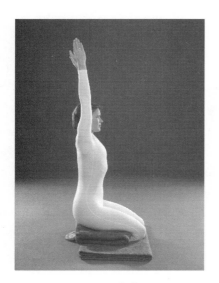

**Photo 8.3**

Reach back, and pull the flesh of your buttocks diagonally back. Rest your hands on your thighs. Press your sitz bones down as you inhale and lengthen your spine up all the way through the crown of your head. Press your shoulder blades into your back, and lift your chest. Keep your chin parallel to the floor (Photo 8.1).

Soften your eyes. Breathe evenly. Move into the world of sensation, where everything is new.

Stretch your arms out to your sides at shoulder height. Rotate your arms and palms to face the ceiling. On an inhalation, stretch your arms up overhead. Feel your arms moving through space. Move with awareness, not out of habit (Photo 8.2).

If possible, bring your palms together and interlace your thumbs. If this is too difficult, keep your arms shoulder-width apart and hold a belt between your hands. Inhale and draw your inner arms up, and press your outer arms in. Keeping your thumbs interlaced or holding the belt, stretch up from your rib cage through your fingertips. Soften your belly, and move your waist back over your hips.

Hold this posture for five to ten breaths. Feel each new breath recharge you with fresh energy. Feel each new breath lift and lengthen your spine even more.

To release, slowly stretch your arms out to your sides and down with awareness. Rest your hands on your thighs. Softly close your eyes; quiet your thinking mind; feel your newly created shape.

Repeat the posture, changing the interlacing of your thumbs. Then release your legs, and stretch them out in front of you.

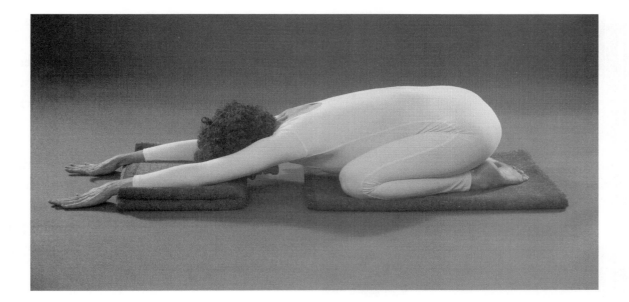

# Extended Child Posture

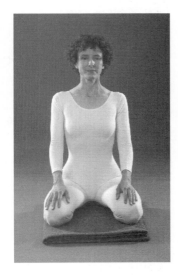

Sit on your heels as in the beginning of Seated Mountain Posture (see Photo 8.1). Keeping your big toes together, move your knees apart just a little wider than your hips (Photo 9.1).

Keep your buttocks down on your heels or on a blanket. Walk your hands forward, shoulder-width apart, and extend your trunk forward and down. Rest your forehead on the floor. Your torso should fit snugly between your thighs.

**Photo 9.1**

If you cannot bring your forehead to the floor, rest your forehead on a blanket and stretch your arms forward, up and over the blanket (Photo 9.2). Alternatively, you can fold your arms and rest them on the blanket.

On an inhalation, keeping your buttocks down on your heels, lengthen your waist, chest, and arms forward.

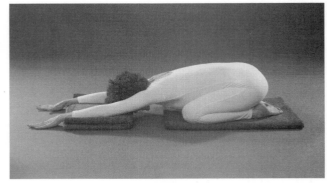

If you cannot bring your buttocks to your heels, place a blanket between your thighs and your calves, wedged up to the inner creases of your knees (Photo 9.3–9.4).

**Photo 9.2**

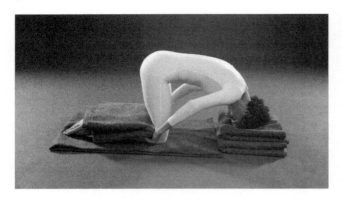

**Photo 9.3**

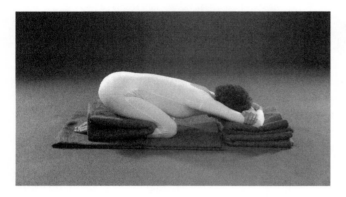

**Photo 9.4**

Hold the posture for five to ten breaths. On each exhalation, release your spine forward and down. Soften your belly. Soften your eyes and the back of your throat. Draw your senses of perception inward. Notice what feels new.

To come up, walk your hands back to the floor beside your knees, and then press your hands into the floor to lift yourself up to a sitting position on your heels. Compare how you feel now with how you felt at the beginning of the posture.

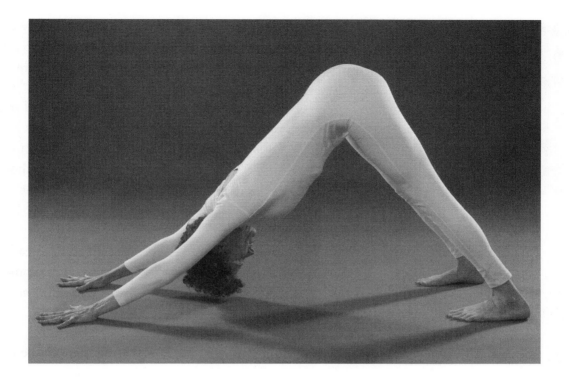

# Downward Dog Posture

Begin on your hands and knees. Walk your hands out about a foot in front of your shoulders, shoulder-width apart. Spread the palms of your hands, and spread your fingers apart. Press firmly into the thumb and index-finger side of your hands.

Press your hands down and straighten your arms. Lift your feet, and come onto the underside of your toes. Move your feet out a little wider than hip-width (Photo 10.1).

Press your hands and feet into the floor. On an exhalation, lift your knees off the floor, raising your hips up and back. As your hips are lifting, stretch your arms and legs to lengthen your spine up and back. Straighten your arms, straighten your legs, and lift your hips higher.

Keep stretching your arms as you press your shoulder blades into your back and lengthen the sides of your trunk up toward your hips. Take your

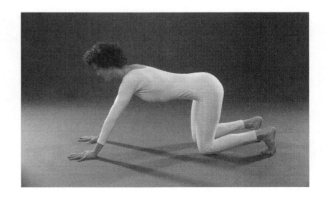

**Photo 10.1**

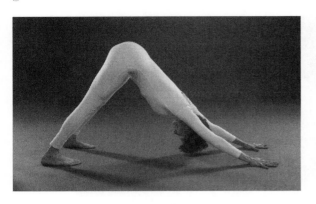

**Photo 10.2**

spine into your body, instead of rounding your back up toward the ceiling. Press the front of your thighs back to help lengthen your spine even more.

Bring your weight into your heels, and stretch your heels back and down. Eventually, you can press them into the floor. Release the back of your neck, and let your head hang down. Your body should be in the shape of a triangle, with your hips at the top of the triangle (Photo 10.2).

Involve yourself with this posture for five to ten breaths, breathing steadily and evenly. On each inhalation, stretch your arms and legs to lengthen your spine more. On each exhalation, release old ways of thinking and moving, and immerse yourself in what is happening now.

When you are ready to release, bend your knees and bring them to the floor. Place the tops of your feet on the floor, and lower your buttocks to your heels. Take your knees apart, and extend your trunk forward into Extended Child Posture (see this chapter, Photos 9.1–9.4). Be here for a few breaths, and let waves of renewal wash over you.

---

### BACK-BENDS

Many people roll their shoulders forward and collapse their chest while doing daily activities. Sitting at a desk, driving a car, cooking a meal, or nursing a baby are a few of a long list of daily activities that reinforce the habitual posture of rolled shoulders and closed chest. Emotional states such as sadness or fear also reinforce forward-collapsed postures. Unlocking habits needs conscious attention. Back-bends such as Locust Posture and Cobra Posture teach you to change your habits. In back-bends, you learn to roll your shoulders in a nonhabitual direction—back and down, away from your ears. You learn to move your spine in new ways, drawing it into your body to support your opening chest and heart.

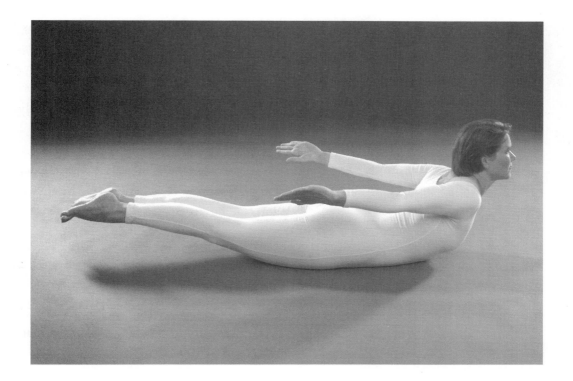

# Locust Posture

### Stage One

Lie down on your belly. Bring your arms down by your sides with your palms facing up. Place your chin on the floor. Extend your legs back, feet together, toes pointed. Press the tops of your feet down into the floor, and stretch and straighten your legs (Photo 11.1).

On an inhalation, press your tailbone down and in, and extend your spine forward. On an exhalation, lift your head, shoulders, chest, and arms up from the floor, arms parallel to the floor. Look forward as you stretch your arms back toward your feet, palms facing up, and lift your chest up even more (Photo 11.2).

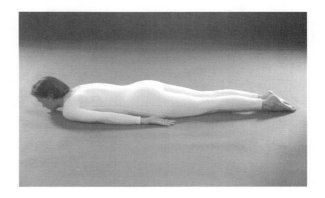

**Photo 11.1**

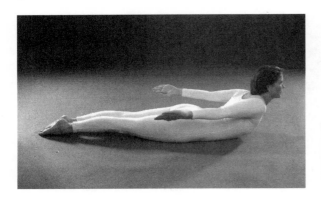

**Photo 11.2**

Hold this stage for three to five breaths. On your inhalations, stretch your arms and legs, lift your chest, and extend your spine. On your exhalations, relax your face and eyes and gather your focus inward. Breathe evenly, and participate fully in creating this new form.

To release, exhale and come down, placing your chin on the floor. Relax your arms beside your body, palms facing up. Soften your eyes and your face.

Repeat this stage of the posture a few times.

## Stage Two

Begin as in Stage One: on your belly, arms down by your sides, palms facing up, chin on the floor, feet together, toes pointed. Press the tops of your feet down into the floor, and stretch and straighten your legs.

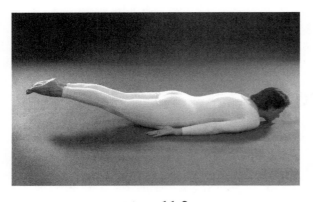

**Photo 11.3**

On an inhalation, contract your buttocks and lift your straight legs up off the floor. Stretch your legs back and up as you hold this stage for three to five breaths, breathing evenly. Relax your face and eyes and focus inward (Photo 11.3).

To release, lower your legs back to the floor and rest there. Repeat this stage of the posture a few times, moving with awareness.

## Stage Three

Begin again on your belly. Now continue by putting the two previous stages together. On an inhalation, contract your buttocks and lift your legs and chest off the floor. Stretch your arms and legs back as you extend your trunk forward and lift your chest up (Photo 11.4). Soften your eyes, relax your face, and look forward. Be in this posture for three to five breaths. Feel your spine moving in a new way, and open your heart.

To release, exhale, come down, and rest on the floor. Bring your arms down by the sides of your body, and rest on one side of your face. By moving out of habitual forms and moving into new shapes, you are opening your field of perception to see the world anew.

Repeat this stage of the posture one or two more times.

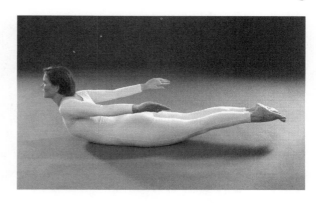

**Photo 11.4**

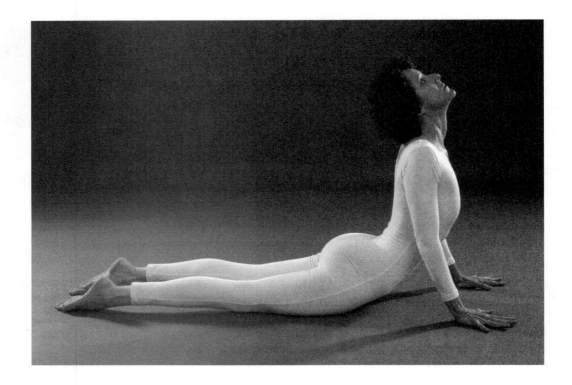

# Cobra Posture

Lie on your belly, legs together, toes pointed, and place your chin on the floor. Place your hands underneath your shoulders, palms down. Spread the palms of your hands, and spread and stretch your fingers apart.

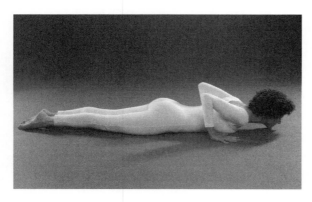

**Photo 12.1**

Bring your upper arms and elbows in toward the sides of your body, and move your shoulder blades down your back. Press your tailbone toward the floor, and slightly squeeze your buttocks. Press the tops of your feet down, and stretch and straighten your legs (Photo 12.1).

Keeping your legs extended, inhale to lift your head and shoulders off the floor without putting any weight on your hands. Look forward, press your shoulder blades into your back, and lift your chest up (Photo 12.2). Take a few breaths here.

Keeping your pubic bone on the floor, inhale and gently press your hands into the floor to lift your chest and belly up from the floor. Lengthen the front of your

spine forward as you rise up. Press your shoulder
blades into your back and expand and lift your
chest upward.

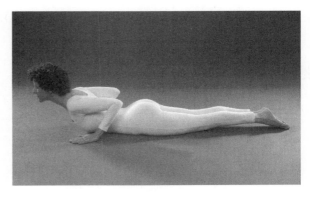

**Photo 12.2**

If you feel any compression in your lower back,
do not straighten your arms completely. Instead,
continue to work on all the actions of the posture,
coming up as high as you can without compression.
Gradually work toward straightening your arms.

Keep your arms hugged in close to your body.
Keep moving your shoulders down away from your
ears. Press your back ribs in to lift your chest higher,
and arch your spine. Finally, take your head back
and look up (Photo 12.3).

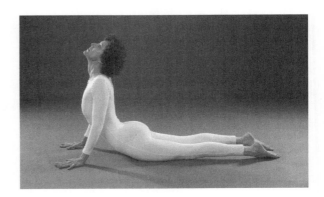

**Photo 12.3**

Open up in this posture for three to five
breaths. Continue extending your legs back as
you open your heart up. Relax your face and eyes,
breathe evenly, and feel your new shape.

To release, bend your elbows and come down
slowly, with awareness, extending your spine forward as you lie back down. Rest on your belly for
a few breaths with your arms down by your sides.
Repeat the posture two or three times. Rest for a
few breaths between repetitions.

After your final repetition, press your palms down into the floor and come up
onto your hands and knees. Lower your buttocks to your heels. Keep your toes
together; move your knees apart; gently extend your trunk and spine forward into a
relaxed Extended Child Posture (see this chapter, Photos 9.1–9.4). Let your elbows
drop to the floor. Soften your face and throat, and rest for a few minutes. Notice
how you feel. In this moment, in every moment, God is renewing your whole body.
With this practice of attentiveness to your whole self, the blessing of renewal is a
reality you can now sense and feel.

# Leaving Egypt

## יציאת מצרים

MANY PEOPLE ARE FAMILIAR with the story of the Jewish people's exodus from Egypt. Far fewer realize that it is also, right now, an ongoing story of personal liberation from limitation, pain, and trouble.

In Hebrew, the word *Egypt* contains the words for "narrow straits" and "water." It evokes layers of meaning about limitation and freedom. Leaving Egypt is therefore more than just a historical event or tribal memory of leaving slavery in a geographical place called Egypt. It is a paradigm for personal experience of release from trouble of all kinds, a release into new possibilities.

In this very moment, you too can leave Egypt. Yoga teaches you ways to actively participate, posture by posture, breath by breath, and moment by moment in leaving Egypt, making it your own story.

## What Is Your Egypt?

Take a moment to consider your life, your story. What troubles or limitations do you face this very moment, this very day? What bondage, internal or external, are you experiencing? All of the narrow straits in your life can be understood as your Egypt. Do you see any possibilities for expansion and release? Can you find a way to leave your Egypt? Torah and yoga can help.

## Torah Yoga for Leaving Egypt

Out of the darkness of Egyptian slavery, the Jewish nation is birthed through the parting waters of the Reed Sea into the light of freedom. This light shines like the light of a new first day of creation, particularly after the darkness and death of the plagues in Egypt which were like a return to the original chaos. How amazing that the rabbis consider this miraculous drama to be the seed that contains all future liberations![1]

Although the story began in Egypt long ago, the rabbis teach that it does not end there. People's lives throughout history are considered part of the ongoing exodus from Egypt. Your life in this moment is an essential part of the story. Your freedom can be found in this story. Because the liberation from Egypt is ongoing, the Torah says many times: "I am God who *is bringing* you out of the land of Egypt" (as in Exodus 6:7, for example) rather than "*who brought* you out of the land of Egypt."

As it says in the Haggadah, the text read, discussed, studied, and sometimes even acted out on the first night of Passover: "In every generation, a person must see himself as if he personally left Egypt." Now is the time to see yourself in this ancient and ever evolving story.

Leaving Egypt is the movement from narrow to expansive places. Every place you are tight, constricted, or in pain is your own personal Egypt. You join the exodus from Egypt when you discover areas of tension and release them. Yoga teaches you how to leave Egypt.

### Liberating Your Mind

In Kabbalah, the story of leaving Egypt is the story of expanding consciousness. *Egypt* is **móchin d'kátnut** (Aramaic for "small mind"). *Leaving Egypt* is **móchin d'gádlut** (Aramaic for "large mind"). You are in Egypt when your mind is contracted. Expanding your mind is the way out of Egypt. But how do you expand your mind? First of all, where exactly is your mind?

The well-acclaimed modern healer and physician Deepak Chopra says that your body is a river of intelligence and information. In other words, your mind is not restricted to the cells of your brain; your intelligence is coursing through all the cells of your body.

Jewish sources also teach that your body is a field of conscious, even divine, intelligence. Jewish mystics teach that there are ten aspects of divine consciousness called **sfirót** (measures). Seven of them are connected to specific areas of the body.

According to the Jewish mystics, then, your mind is located throughout your body. (I am not going further into the subject of the **sfirót** in this book. Suffice it to say that they are a spiritual reality map for all of creation, the underlying theoretical framework for all of Jewish mysticism.)

Yoga, as well, teaches that your whole body is a field of consciousness. Yoga is a technique for waking up the river of intelligence and information, the consciousness, in all the parts of your body. Because your body is your mind, when you stretch, lengthen, breathe, and release into expanded inner spaces, you are expanding your consciousness. Opening your body *is* opening your mind.

## Liberating Your Body

The many parts of your body exist in various degrees of contracted and expanded consciousness. Those parts in expanded consciousness are open to unlimited possibilities. Those parts in contracted consciousness are more closed and limited. Often, people are not even aware of these closed and limited parts. Jewish tradition teaches that the worst part of the exile in Egypt was that the Jews were not even aware that they were in exile. Becoming conscious of your narrow places is the first step in releasing them. Yoga postures are designed to find both conscious and unconscious constrictions that you hold in your body.

Yoga is an ongoing journey of movement from narrow places to expanded possibilities. It teaches you to stretch beyond what you think your limits are. Repeatedly I have witnessed students who are astonished and delighted as their bodies move in ways they did not think were possible.

Your body wants to open. Yoga provides opportunities for opening in a gentle, loving way. Through breath and movement, you learn to release yourself, cell by cell, from your narrow straits. You may enter a yoga class full of tensions and troubles, and come out as free-flowing as the wide-open sea.

## Liberating Your Emotions

Leaving Egypt through yoga is not simply a physical release. Your body stores emotions, memories, and experiences in its very cells. Pain or trauma may manifest in a tense belly. Anger may be held in tight shoulders or clenched fists. Sadness may be lying curled up in your forward-rolling shoulders. When you encounter places in your body with yoga, you encounter your life experiences. When you open your chest, you may release a stream of tears or a burst of laughter. When you stretch your legs into a vulnerably open posture, old memories of fear or love may suddenly appear to you.

## Liberating Your Soul

Rav Kook writes of the desire of the soul to be free of all narrowness and limitation: "Expanses, expanses, expanses divine my soul craves. Do not confine me in any physical or spiritual cage. My soul sails in the heavenly expanse."[2]

Yoga is like a winged ship taking you on your own divine voyage from your narrow straits to a sea of heavenly expansiveness. With yoga, explore the opportunity to set sail for the open sea from all the different places within you. In practicing the postures, experience leaving Egypt.

##  Torah Study for Leaving Egypt

On a literal level, leaving Egypt is the Torah's account of God freeing the Jewish people from their slavery in Egypt. However, it is also a spiritual concept, the most pervasive spiritual idea reverberating through all of Torah and Jewish practice.

### Leaving Egypt in Torah

Throughout Torah, there are repeated lessons and reminders of leaving Egypt. For example, in Deuteronomy 16:3, we are told to remember leaving Egypt every day: "Remember the day you left Egypt *all* the days of your life." Actually, because the passage says "*all* the days of your life" and not simply "the days of your life," the Mishnah teaches that you should remember leaving Egypt in both the days *and nights* of your life. The Mishnah then expands this further. It teaches that "days of your life" refers to the days of your life in this world; "*all* the days of your life" includes the days of your life in the world to come (when Messiah comes).[3] Leaving Egypt is so significant that, whether it is day or night, this world or the next, it must be remembered.

The first of the Ten Commandments says: "I am the Lord, your God, who brought you out of the land of Egypt, the house of slavery" (Exodus 20:2; Deuteronomy 5:6). It does *not* say, "I am the Lord, your God, who created you." According to Sfat Emet, this teaches that leaving Egypt is more essential than creation itself.[4] He also teaches that leaving Egypt has meaning not just every day but even every moment of our lives. "The truth is that at *every moment*, for *every person* of Israel, there is [we are faced with] *Egypt*. Therefore we remember *leaving Egypt* every day."[5] How do we remember leaving Egypt? It is woven like a recurring pattern into the fabric of traditional Jewish practice.

## Leaving Egypt in Prayers

Leaving Egypt appears throughout the traditional daily prayers. "I am the Lord your God who brought you out of the land of Egypt" is recited morning and evening.[6] Sabbaths and holidays are all called reminders of leaving Egypt in the blessing over the wine that ushers in these holy times.[7]

On the first evening of Passover, Jewish families gather to celebrate the exodus from Egypt. Traditionally, they read the Haggadah at this time. According to the Haggadah itself, simply reading the text is not enough. One must be so involved that one comes to see oneself in the story. One must personally experience leaving Egypt.

## Mystery and Meaning in the Hebrew Letters

What deeper meaning gives the story of leaving Egypt the honor of being the constant heartbeat of Jewish life? How is this ancient story personally relevant every moment of our day-to-day lives?

The Hebrew letters *mem, tsádi, resh, yud,* and *mem sofít* spell the word *mitsráyim* (Egypt). These five letters contain teachings, literal and mystical, about the ongoing significance of leaving Egypt.

All Hebrew letters are consonants—there are no written vowels in the Torah. The same letters can make different words depending on the vowel sounds used. The same five Hebrew letters that spell *mitsráyim* (Egypt)—with different vowel sounds supplied—spell the word *metsarím* (narrow straits). Leaving Egypt can thus be understood as leaving narrow straits.

Another careful look at the letters of the word *mitsráyim* reveals more of its secret meaning and power. The second and third letters, *tsádi* and *resh,* spell the word *tsar* (narrow). The word *tsar* also has the connotations of limitation, trouble, and pain—like the word *tsúris* in Yiddish. The surrounding letters—*mem, yud,* and *mem sofít*—spell the word *máyim* (water). Water flows and expands to fill whatever space it is given. It is a symbol of unlimited possibilities. It is a harbinger of new life.[8]

With this letter-by-letter understanding, we see that this one Hebrew word contains a magnificent spiritual teaching. *Egypt* is *tsar* surrounded by *máyim:* narrowness, trouble, limitation, and pain surrounded by flowing, expansive possibilities for new life. *Leaving Egypt* therefore means going even beyond the world of contraction and expansion, narrowness and expansiveness, to a place we have no name for yet. The psalmist says, "From the narrow places I called out, and I was answered in the expanded places of God" (Psalms 118:5).

*Leaving Egypt* is a concept worthy of remembering all the days of our lives because—generally, whether simple or profound—some aspect of *tsar* (narrowness) is in our lives every day. You can join the ongoing story of the exodus from Egypt every moment, as you move from breath to breath and from choice to choice through the troubles and narrow passages in your life.

*Máyim* (water) is the symbol of expansion, potential, and new life. It sounds almost like the two Hebrew words *ma im* (what if). Take a moment to sense the expansive waters surrounding the troubles in your life. Hear the water whispering to you the words: "What if . . .?" Imagine good and beautiful things. What if I . . .?" Imagine you can.

## Yoga Practice for Leaving Egypt

With yoga, you can personally experience leaving Egypt. While in your postures, notice any areas that feel tight or constricted. Call out from those places. After each posture, appreciate any inner responses of release and expansiveness. Feel your breath flow and let your practice take you to the open sea.

Press your left thigh back and tuck your right buttock under. Stretch your right inner thigh from your groin outward to your knee (Photo 13.1).

On an exhalation, extend your trunk out over your right leg, bringing your right fingertips down to the floor or to a block beside your right ankle. Place your left hand on your hip. Continue to tuck your right buttock under, and stretch your right inner thigh from your groin to your knee.

Stretch your left arm straight up, palm facing forward (Photo 13.2). Inhale and lengthen your spine from your tailbone through the crown of your head.

Rotate your left arm so that your palm faces to the right. On an exhalation, extend your left arm out over your left ear.

Press the outer edge of your left foot into the floor, and stretch the entire left side of your body from your left heel all the way out through the tips of your left fingers. Press your shoulder blades into your back, and open your chest.

Turn the front of your trunk from right to left. Press your right knee back into your right elbow, and press your right buttock forward. Roll the left side of your trunk up and away from the floor to keep the front of your trunk facing forward (Photo 13.3). Finally, turn your head to look up toward the ceiling.

Be engaged in this posture for three to five breaths, breathing evenly. Breathe into your expanding body. Expand what you believe is possible for yourself.

To come out of the posture, press your left foot firmly into the floor and stretch your left arm up. Press both heels into the floor. On an inhalation, straighten your right leg and lift your trunk upright. Turn your feet back to center, and step or jump them back together. Take a moment to drink in the benefits of this posture.

Repeat this posture on the other side.

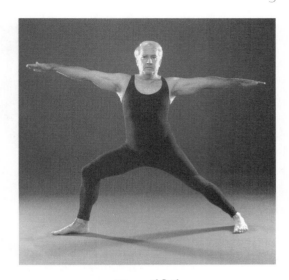

**Photo 13.1**

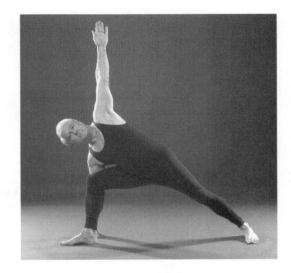

**Photo 13.2**

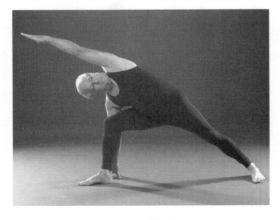

**Photo 13.3**

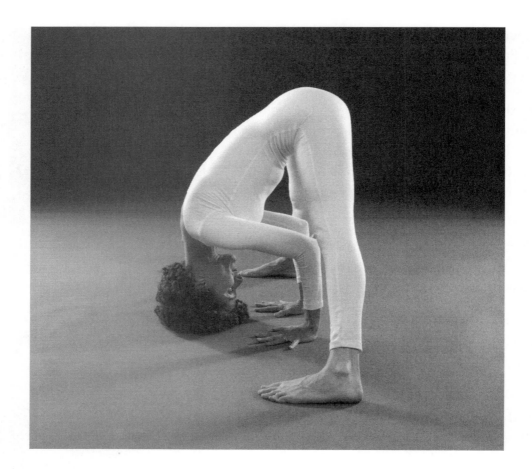

# Wide Legs Standing Forward Bend

### Stage One

Stand in Mountain Posture (see Chapter One, Photos 2.1–2.2).

Bring your hands to your hips. On an inhalation, step or jump your feet four and a half to five feet apart. Turn your toes in slightly, your heels out. Press your feet firmly into the floor and stretch your legs upward.

With your hands on your hips, draw your elbows back behind you and toward each other (Photo 14.1). Lift and open your chest.

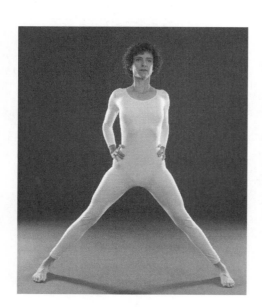

**Photo 14.1**

On an exhalation, extend your trunk forward and place your fingertips on the floor or on blocks underneath your shoulders. Straighten your arms and lengthen them.

Press your feet into the floor, and stretch your legs up. Keeping your hips aligned over your heels, press the fronts of your thighs back toward the thighbones, and extend your spine and chest forward.

Turn your inner arms forward. Lift your head and look forward. Press your shoulder blades into your back, and roll your collarbone up toward the ceiling. Make your back concave by taking your back ribs in and lifting the front of your chest up (Photo 14.2). This is the concave part of the posture. Stay in this position for three to five breaths, lengthening your spine forward.

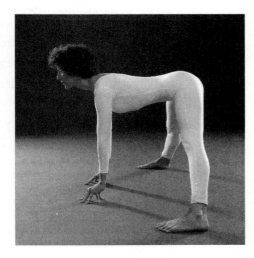

**Photo 14.2**

### Stage Two

On an exhalation, walk your hands back, placing them between your feet, shoulder-width apart, fingers facing forward. Bend your elbows, and have your forearms parallel to each other.

On an exhalation, extend your trunk down toward the floor. Rest the crown of your head on the floor or on a block between your hands (Photo 14.3). Lift your shoulder blades up away from your ears. Keep the weight of your body on your feet, not your head, and stretch your legs up. Keep your hips aligned over your heels.

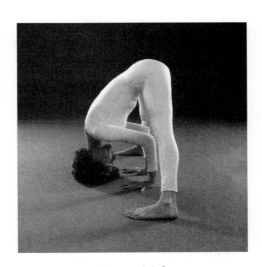

**Photo 14.3**

Be in this position for three to five breaths, breathing evenly. Focus your attention on the sensations in your body. Draw yourself deep enough into the posture to meet places of tightness, constriction, or resistance. In your body, now, you have the opportunity to leave Egypt. Do not force or strain your way through your narrow straits. Breathe and wait for the gates to open.

To come out of the posture, walk your hands forward and come back to the concave part of the posture. Heel-toe your feet in toward each other once or twice. Straighten your legs, and press your feet into the floor. Place your hands on your hips. Inhale and lead with your chest to come up to standing.

Jump or step your feet back together. Soften and take time to feel the effects of the posture.

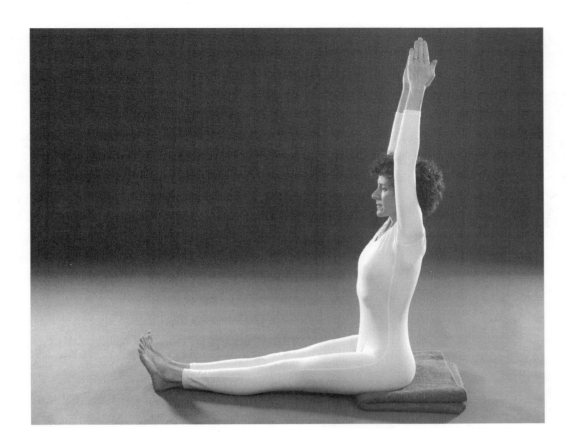

# Staff Posture

Sit on the floor with your legs extended out in front of you. If your lower back pushes out to the back, sit on a firm blanket. Use your hands to pull the flesh of your buttocks out to the sides and diagonally back, and sit up on the tips of your sitz bones.

Join the inner edges of your legs and feet, and stretch them forward. Press out through the heels and the balls of your feet. Press your thighs down toward the floor.

Bring your hands down and back by the sides of your hips, fingers facing forward. Press the palms of your hands into the floor or the blanket. On an inhalation, press your hands down, stretch your arms and legs, and lift your chest and spine upward.

Press your thighs firmly down into the floor, and inhale to lift your spine even more. Lengthen the front of your trunk up to your collarbone.

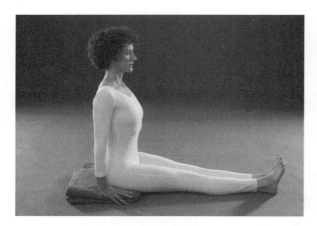

**Photo 15.1**

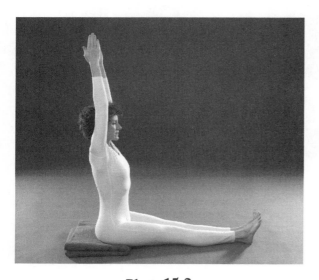

**Photo 15.2**

Roll your upper arms and shoulders back, and press your shoulder blades into your body. Keep your ears over your shoulders and your chin parallel to the floor (Photo 15.1).

On an inhalation, extend your arms out to your sides at shoulder height, palms facing down. Rotate your arms so that your palms face up. On an inhalation, lift your chest, and raise your arms up over your head, palms facing each other (Photo 15.2).

Breathing evenly, stay in this posture for three to five breaths, continually pressing your thighs firmly into the floor and lifting your spine and chest up. Feel the sensations of this stretch. Relax your face, your eyes, and your breath.

To release, lower your arms down to your sides and come to a cross-legged position. Notice how you feel.

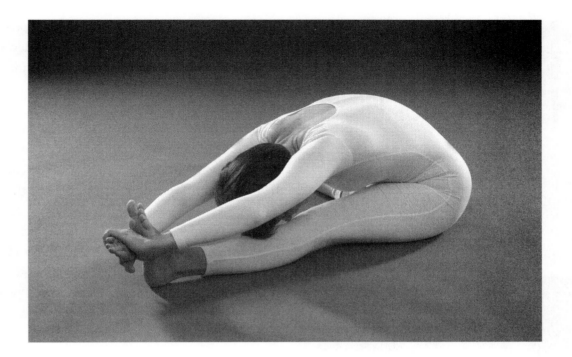

# Head Beyond Knee Forward Bend

## Stage One

Begin in Staff Posture (see this chapter, Photo 15.1) with your legs stretched out in front of you, arms down by your sides. Sit on a blanket if you need to so that you can straighten your lower back.

Turn your right knee out to the side. Holding the inside of your right knee from on top, bend and pull your knee back as far as you can while keeping both hips facing forward.

Bring your right heel to the top of your inner right thigh, right toes touching your inner left thigh, sole of your right foot facing up. Bring your right knee to the floor, or place a blanket underneath your right knee for support.

Press your left thigh downward, and extend out through the heel and ball of your left foot. Place the fingertips of your right hand on the floor in front of you and the fingertips of your left hand on the floor behind you.

Pressing your left leg to the floor and your right knee back and down, press into your hands to lift your spine and turn your torso from right to left, so that

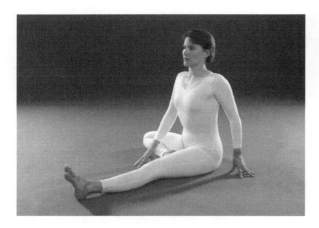

**Photo 16.1**

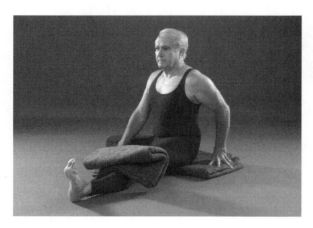

**Photo 16.2**

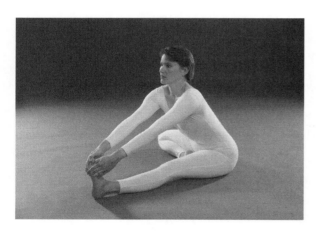

**Photo 16.3**

your torso faces over your left leg. Inhale, press your sitz bones down, and lengthen up both sides of your torso evenly as you turn your trunk more from right to left (Photos 16.1–16.2).

Keep your spine lengthening up as you stretch your arms forward and hold the sides of your left foot with your hands; alternately, wrap a belt under the ball of your foot and hold the sides of the belt.

Press your left thigh and right knee firmly into the floor, and straighten your arms (Photo 16.3). Move your back ribs in, and inhale to lengthen the front of your spine. Lift your chest and roll your collarbone up. Relax your eyes and look straight ahead of you.

Breathe evenly into areas that feel tight, and give yourself time to arrive fully into this concave part of the posture. Whether this is your first experience in this posture or you have been practicing it for years, there is an opportunity here and now for more freedom, more expansion.

## Stage Two

To go further, bend and lift your elbows up and out to the sides and bend at your hips as you lengthen your torso forward over your left leg. Turn the right side of your torso down, and see that you are lengthening the right and left sides of your torso evenly. Bring your forehead down to your shin or to a blanket or bolster placed on top of your leg (Photo 16.4).

If you need to, be sure to use adequate props so that your forehead is supported. Resting your forehead quiets your brain. This makes a difference in how well you can relax and release into the stretch. Props can assist you in leaving Egypt.

Continue to press your left leg, right thigh, and knee firmly to the floor and extend your spine forward. Move slowly with finely tuned awareness as you navigate your way into this stretch.

When you are well extended over your leg, you can switch your hand position. Turn your palms to face away from you. Hold the back of your right hand or wrist with your left hand, and place the backs of your hands on the ball of your foot. Press your hands into your foot to lengthen your spine over your leg (Photo 16.5).

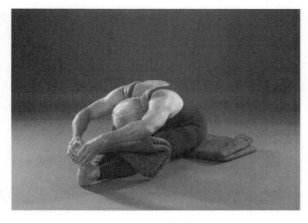

**Photo 16.4**

Immerse yourself in this posture for three to five breaths. Continue to turn your right side down so that your right and left sides are stretching evenly over your extending leg. Quiet your brain; relax your face and eyes; meet resistance with breath and patience. Notice when tightness dissolves into the surrounding expanse, and then move deeper into the posture.

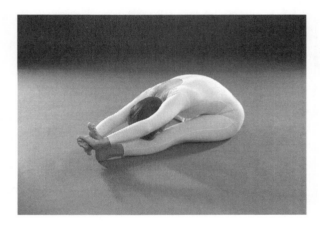

**Photo 16.5**

To release, press into the floor with your left leg and rise up to the concave part of the posture. Stretch your spine forward, lift your collarbone, and look forward. Then inhale and lift your torso all the way up.

Soften and receive the benefits of this posture. Every posture is a gateway to inner space. Take a moment to experience your own inner spaciousness.

Repeat the posture on the other side.

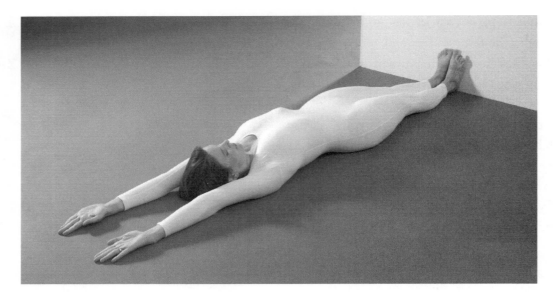

**Photo 17.1**

# Reclining Mountain Posture

Lie on your back with the soles of your feet against the base of a wall, arms down by your sides. Join the inner edges of your legs and feet. Stretch and straighten your legs, and press them down toward the floor as you press your feet into the wall.

On an inhalation, stretch your arms up to the ceiling, shoulder-width apart, palms facing each other. Reach up toward the ceiling; then inhale again, and extend your arms to the floor above your head, palms facing up.

Press your feet firmly into the wall and stretch your arms, lengthening your spine away from your legs. If you moved away from the wall when you brought your arms up, slide in closer so that your heels are firmly in contact with the wall. Inhale and gently lengthen the back of your neck away from your shoulders (Photo 17.1).

Relax your face and eyes as you continue to actively energize and lengthen your legs and spine for five to seven breaths. Gaze inward, and feel the intelligence of your body-mind waking up.

On an exhalation, keep lengthening your spine away from your legs as you raise your arms up toward the ceiling; then lower them down by your sides.

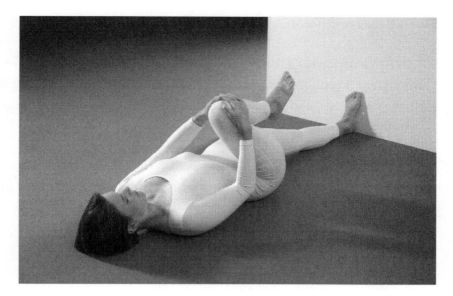

**Photo 18.1**

# Knee-to-Chest Posture

Lie on your back with your feet against the base of a wall. Press your left heel firmly into the wall and bend your right knee. With your hands clasped on top of your knee, bring your knee toward your chest.

Keep pressing your left foot firmly into the wall as you press your left leg down toward the floor. Stretch and lengthen your left leg.

Using your arms, gently pull your right knee in toward your chest and soften your right groin. Move your outer right thigh and buttock toward the wall to lengthen the right side of your waist (Photo 18.1). Feel the subtle ways you can make more space in your body.

Lengthen your spine away from your legs. Relax your shoulders, and open and broaden your chest.

Soften your face and eyes and the back of your throat, and breathe evenly in this posture for five to seven breaths. This posture is excellent for releasing tension from your lower back. Feel your lower back relaxing.

To release, straighten your right leg and join your legs back together. Adjust your legs and buttocks, making sure your heels are again pressing into the wall and that your spine is aligned in the center of your body.

Repeat the posture on the other side.

After performing the posture on both sides, bend both knees in toward your chest, keeping the back of your pelvis on the floor. Hold your knees with your hands, and gently pull both knees in as you soften your groin and lengthen your spine.

Relax all the muscles and the skin of your face. Relax your shoulders. Quiet your thoughts, and breathe evenly in this posture for five to seven breaths.

To release, lower your feet to the floor, and rest there.

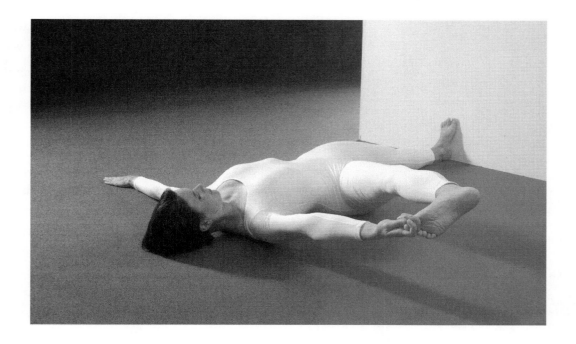

# Reclining Leg Stretch

### Stage One—Leg Straight Up

Lie on your back with the inner edge of your legs and feet joined together and your feet firmly pressed into the base of a wall.

Press your left leg down and stretch it toward the wall while you bend your right knee, as in the Knee to Chest Posture (see this chapter, Photo 18.1). Move your outer right thigh and buttock toward the wall while you lengthen your spine away from your legs.

Make a ring grip around your right big toe, using the thumb, index, and middle fingers of your right hand (Photo 19.1).

On an exhalation, straighten your right leg up toward the ceiling (Photo 19.2). If you cannot straighten your right leg while holding your right big toe, place a strap around the ball of your right foot. Hold the strap with both hands, and straighten your right leg up (Photo 19.3).

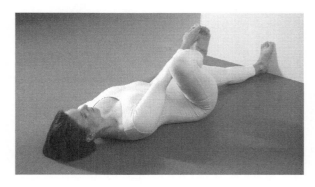

**Photo 19.1**

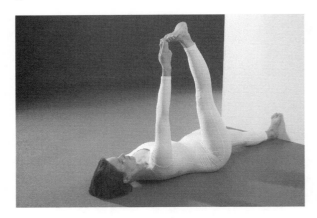

**Photo 19.2**

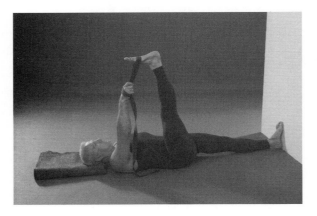

**Photo 19.3**

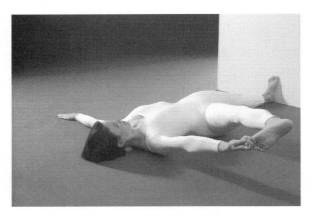

**Photo 19.4**

Stretch your leg until you come to a place of tension or resistance, a narrow strait. Relax your face, and direct your breath to the tight area. Spend a few breaths tending to your tightness with breath and patience. Follow the cues of your body on your way out of Egypt.

Press the front of your right thigh back toward the wall, and press up into the heel and ball of your right foot. Press your left thigh down toward the floor and extend your left leg, pressing your heel firmly into the wall.

If you feel your body opening and wanting a deeper stretch, then go further. You do not always have to go further. Where you are right now, there are opportunities for release and expansion.

Maintain your quiet focus and stay active in this stretch, breathing evenly, for five to seven breaths.

## Stage Two—Leg to Side

If you are not using a belt, continue holding your right big toe with your ring grip. If you are using a belt, reach up as high as you can with your right hand toward your right foot, and hold the belt with your right hand. Stretch your left arm out to your side at shoulder height, palm facing down.

On an exhalation, lower your right leg out to the side and down, drawing it up toward the line of your right shoulder, while you press your left thigh and buttock down toward the floor to prevent rolling to the right. Take your right leg only as far as you can, while still keeping your left thigh and buttock down. Breathe your way into this stretch.

Open your chest, and stretch your left arm further to the left. Stretch your right inner thigh further to the right while keeping your left shoulder, buttock, and thigh pressed down (Photos 19.4–19.5).

Quiet your thinking mind and any goal-oriented aspirations, and attend to the intelligence of your body-mind. Does your body want to move deeper into the stretch? Each time you meet a new edge, a new momentary limitation, wait there and breathe. When you feel the edge soften, move into the expanding space.

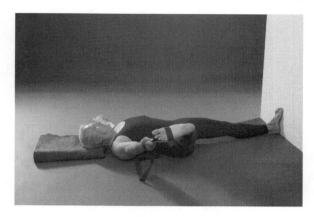

**Photo 19.5**

Soften your face and eyes and the back of your throat. Navigate the waters of possibility with gentleness and patience. Stay in this position for three to five breaths. With each inhalation, refocus your attention inward; with each exhalation, relax into the stretch.

To release, on an inhalation, raise your right leg back up to the Leg Straight Up position. On an exhalation, bend your right knee, remove the belt, and straighten your right leg. Bring your legs and feet back together. Realign your spine. Then repeat the posture on the other side.

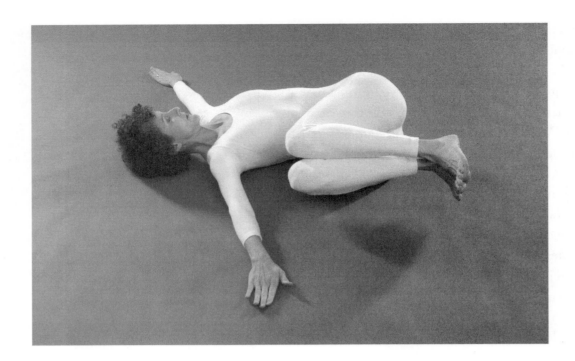

# Reclining Twist

Lie on your back with your knees bent, arms down by your sides and feet on the floor.

Lift your feet up off the floor, and draw your thighs and knees in toward your belly with your hands. Keeping your knees pulled in toward your belly, stretch your arms out to your sides at shoulder height, palms down on the floor (Photo 20.1).

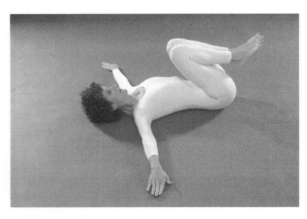

**Photo 20.1**

Continue to actively stretch your left arm, keeping your left shoulder close to the floor, while you lower your legs down to your right, keeping your thighs together and pulled in toward your belly. Lower your bent legs to the right until your knees and feet hover over the floor, knees pointing diagonally up toward your right arm. Lengthen your left thigh so that your left knee stays directly over your right knee.

Draw your belly in toward your spine and twist your torso from right to left, so that your heart faces the ceiling. Lengthen both arms out along the floor, and broaden and expand your chest (Photo 20.2).

Soften your face and eyes as you engage in this twist for three to five breaths. Relax your breathing.

To release, on an exhalation, slowly return to center. Place your feet on the floor and lift your buttocks up slightly to realign your spine in the center of your back. Then lower your buttocks back down and rest. Rest your arms down by your sides.

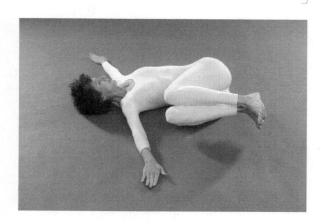

**Photo 20.2**

Twists release tensions in the spine, freeing it up to move more easily. They are also cleansing and revitalizing for your abdominal organs. Take a moment to notice and appreciate the effects of the posture.

Repeat the twist on the second side.

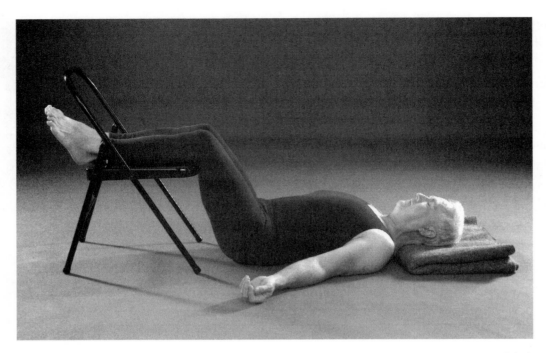

**Photo 21.1**

# Resting with Legs on Chair

Lie on the floor on your back with your head and neck on a folded firm blanket.

Bend your knees, and rest the whole length of your calves up on the seat of a chair. Place your arms down at your sides, and rotate your arms so that your palms face up (Photo 21.1). Relax your arms and hands, letting your fingers curl.

Gently close your eyes and rest here for several minutes. Wriggle your way into a comfortable, supported position; then let your body be still. Relax your forehead, eyes, and the skin on your face. Relax your brain. Let go of any effort. With each exhalation, let tensions dissolve into a surrounding openness. Move inward and quietly observe your inner space.

As your outer body comes to stillness, tune in to the world of subtle vibrations. Feel your soul soaring freely in a great inner expanse.

To release, roll to your right side and lie in the fetal position for a few breaths. Then press into the floor with your hands and come up to sitting.

# The Essential Self

# האני העצמי

AFTER EATING THE FORBIDDEN FRUIT, Adam and Eve hide among the trees in the Garden of Eden (Genesis 3:8). They are hiding from God, of course, but also from themselves. Everyone—in different ways, for different reasons, and at different moments in life—hides like Adam and Eve.

While they are hiding, God calls to Adam: "Where are you?" (Genesis 3:9). Rashi says: "God knows where Adam is. Nevertheless, God calls to Adam in order to enter into conversation with him."[1] God wants Adam to answer with *hinéni* (here I am). In the Torah, Abraham, Jacob, Moses, and Samuel answer *hinéni* when God calls. It is a response expressing total self-presence and readiness to enter into conversation with God.

Yoga is a way to stop hiding—a way to meet and enter into intimate and holy conversation with God and with yourself.

## Where Are You?

Ask yourself, "Where am I?" Listen to your response. Have an unhurried conversation with yourself. Be attentive to all the many aspects of yourself. What are they saying to you right now? Now ask the question again. This time answer with the words "Here I am," keeping in mind all those aspects of yourself that you just conversed with. How do you feel when you respond this way?

**Torah Yoga for the Essential Self**

"Where are you?" This is the first question God asks in the Torah. Adam does not directly answer God's question. He says: "I heard your voice in the garden and I was afraid because I am naked and I hid" (Genesis 3:10). Rav Kook says, "He did not clearly answer the question 'where are you?' because he did not know his own soul, because his true *I-ness* [his essential self], was lost to him."[2]

Adam's lack of self-knowledge, his alienation from self, is the first exile. This primordial exile begins even before Adam and Eve are banished from the Garden of Eden. It is marked by the inability to clearly and openly answer the question "Where are you?"

Yoga is a way to meet and know your essential self. Each posture is an opportunity to connect with yourself and to clearly and openly answer "Here I am " to the question "Where are you?" It is a way home for the self that is in exile.

## Find a Teacher—Learn from Yourself

On your way home to yourself, teachers can be helpful. There are traditions in both the Jewish world and the yoga community that advocate having *one* teacher. So who is the one teacher for you, your final authority?

Torah says: *aséi lechá rav*—usually translated as "Find yourself a teacher."[3] However, *aséi* literally means "make." Therefore, this passage can also mean "Make yourself into a teacher" or even "Make yourself into your own teacher." In other words, *you* must be the one teacher for you. You are the only one who can truly and meaningfully answer the question "Where are you?" Therefore, ultimately, you must be the final authority for yourself.

Learn from teachers, but do not lose your connection to your own wisdom by focusing exclusively on the wisdom of others. Let the teachings you receive from outside sources deepen your connection to yourself and to your own inner knowing. When doing your yoga postures, trust your own intuitions, your own experience—trust yourself. Yoga will clarify your inner wisdom. Listen to your inner guidance. Eventually, your own body-mind-heart-soul will be your greatest teacher.

## Meet and Know Yourself

The first step to knowing yourself is meeting and becoming aware of yourself. Torah teaches: "Greet everyone you meet with a beautiful face."[4] When you meet yourself in a yoga posture, you come face to face with your whole self. On any given day, you are a mysterious blend of your physical, intellectual, emotional, and spiritual aspects. Meet your whole self with a beautiful face of kindness.

Become aware of all the many aspects of yourself. You may sense energy, subtle vibration, heat, or cold. You may feel strong, flexible, tired, or energized. You may discover anger or sadness. You may feel ecstasy and bliss. You may see new colors or interesting shapes. You may feel as though you suddenly drop into water or that you are actually made of vast inner space. You may have a clear memory from your past or receive creative insights.

The Torah says that human beings are created in the image of God (Genesis 1:26). In Hebrew, another way to say God is **ein sof** (no end). Because you are created in the image of **ein sof,** there is no end to what you can discover about yourself. There are an unlimited number of postures in yoga. Each posture is an opportunity to become more conscious that you are created in the image of God. Each posture can bring you home to another aspect of yourself. Use yoga to enter into conversation with your divine and mysterious essence.

 ## Torah Study for the Essential Self

The first exile was the alienation of Adam and Eve from themselves while still in the Garden of Eden. Stories throughout the Torah hint at this existential state of exile. God's first words to Abraham are these: "Go from your land, from your birthplace, from your father's home, to a land that I will show you" (Genesis 12:1). The first two words of this passage in Hebrew, **lech lechá,** are often translated simply as "go." Paying attention to the literal meaning of the second word, **lechá** ("to you" or "for you"), the *Zohar* teaches that these two words mean "go to yourself."[5] God is telling Abraham to go on a journey to himself.

Existential exile also plays a part in the story of Jacob. After his prophetic dream, the Torah says: "And Jacob wakes from his sleep and says, 'Surely God is in this place and **anochí** [I] **lo yadáti** [I did not know]'" (Genesis 28:16). There are abundant commentaries about the apparently superfluous **anochí** (I).[6] One explanation is that "I" is referring to Jacob himself. Jacob realized that, until now, he did not know himself—"And *I,* I did not know." Jacob, awakened by God's presence, awakes as well to an awareness of his essential self. Jacob's comment on his dream expresses an inextricable connection between sensing God and knowing oneself.

### Exile and External Validation

Exile is most commonly understood as banishment from one's native country. In Jewish history, it refers to banishment from the land of Israel. Exile is a recurring motif throughout the Bible and indeed throughout Jewish history to this day. Rav Kook, however, develops the idea that exile is the existential state of alienation from self.[7] He bases his idea on one line from Ezekiel (1:1): "And *I* am in the midst of exile."

Rav Kook hears in Ezekiel's words a link to Adam's state in the garden. He reads this passage with an emphasis on the first word. "'*I* am in the midst of exile'—the *I* is the inner *essential self.*"[8] In other words, the essential self is in exile—it has been banished from its home. Rav Kook continues to describe how, actually, all of creation is in exile from its essential self. The individual as well as the community—and even plants, animals, and inanimate creations like the moon—are in exile from their inner essence.

What causes the essential self to be in exile? One answer is that, in all of creation, exile is a result of relying too much on external sources of information and validation. For example, when does Adam become alienated from his own self? According to Rav Kook, it happens when Adam relies on the knowledge of the snake, a source outside himself, instead of relying on his own knowledge. In another example, Rashi teaches that, originally, the moon and sun were both great lights of equal size. As it compares itself with the sun, the moon becomes dissatisfied. It seeks the glorious title of being the only "king of lights."[9] In response to the moon's lack of satisfaction with itself and desire for a glorious title, God diminishes the moon's light. The moon is exiled from its original fully radiant self when it seeks external validation.

Looking outside of its own essence, the self of all creation goes into exile.

## Education and Loss of Self

Rav Kook writes about the role of some educators in furthering the loss of self. "The 'great' educators come and they only look at external things. They also distract one from knowing the self. They put straw on the fire, they give thirsty ones vinegar to drink; they stuff up minds and hearts with everything that is external to them, and the self is forgotten."[10]

In other words, some educators offer an "external" education that is ultimately not sustaining or satisfying because people are actually hungry and thirsty to know their own selves. Straw does not feed the fire—vinegar does not quench the thirst—of a soul longing to know itself. Being stuffed up with external information leaves the essential self undernourished.

Rav Kook teaches that study can either fan the flames of each unique soul or put out the fire.[11] Sources of information, internal and external, that nourish your unique self are the real fuel for the fire of your soul. They are your satisfying food and thirst-quenching drink.

Rav Kook assures us that the self will return home from exile. With his characteristic optimism, he says, "We will search for ourselves and we will find ourselves."[12]

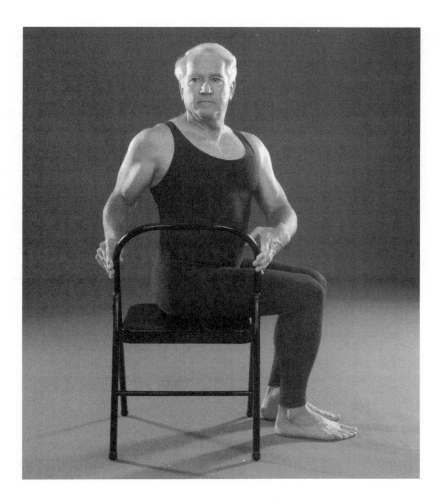

# Chair Twist Posture

For this posture, you need a chair with a flat seat and a backrest.

Sit so that the right side of your body faces the back of the chair. Place your feet on the floor hip-width apart. Your thighs should be parallel to the floor. Place a firm blanket evenly under your feet if you need to, so that your thighs are parallel to the floor.

Pull the flesh of your buttocks out to the sides and diagonally back, and sit evenly on both sides of your buttocks (Photo 22.1). Move your tailbone down, inhale, and lengthen your spine up through the crown of your head.

Begin to turn your torso from left to right. Hold on to the sides of the back of the chair. On inhalations, lengthen your spine even

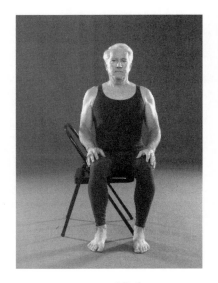

**Photo 22.1**

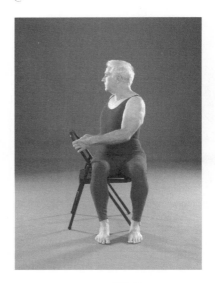

**Photo 22.2**

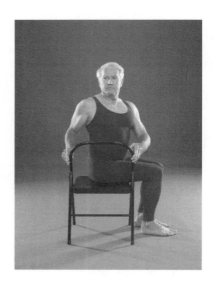

**Photo 22.3**

more, creating space between each vertebra. On exhalations, turn your torso more from left to right. Have your face turned in the same direction your heart is facing (Photo 22.2).

Press firmly into your left buttock so that your left knee does not inch forward. Keep your knees parallel to each other.

Keep your shoulders down away from your ears. Lift your elbows slightly up and out to the sides to broaden your chest and collarbone.

Pull the left side of the chair with your left hand to help you turn the left side of your torso to the right. Keep your left shoulder back.

Push into the right side of the chair with your right hand to turn the right side of your torso further to the right and to move your right shoulder back (Photo 22.3).

For three to five breaths, spiral your way more deeply into the twist, inhaling to lengthen and exhaling to turn. Do not force yourself. Relax your eyes; quiet your thinking mind; let the intelligence of your own body guide you into the twist.

To release, turn slowly back to center.

Repeat the twist on the second side.

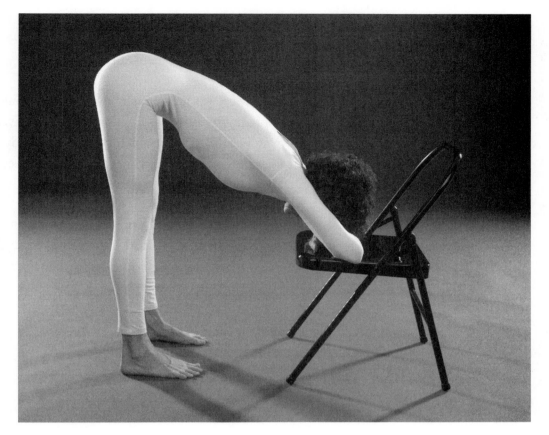

**Photo 23.1**

# Supported Standing Forward Bend with Chair

Place a chair about two feet in front of you, with the seat of the chair facing you. Stand with your feet hip-width apart, toes slightly turned in, heels out. Broaden and lengthen your feet, and spread and stretch your toes. Lift the arches of your feet.

Press your heels into the floor, and stretch your legs up. Lift the fronts of your thighs up to the crease of your groin, and lift and firm your kneecaps. Rotate your upper thighs in toward each other, and press them back to the bone.

Inhale and raise your arms up over your head. Fold your arms and clasp your elbows. Holding your elbows securely, lift your arms up toward the ceiling, lengthening the sides of your torso and rib cage. Lift and expand your chest.

Keep stretching your legs upward, and on an exhalation, bend forward from your hips, bringing your folded arms to the seat of the chair. Rest your forehead on your arms (Photo 23.1). Relax your eyes and quiet your brain.

Continue to actively stretch your legs up, and let your spine passively release into the support of the chair. Be present with yourself in this posture for five to ten breaths. Feel the sensations in your body. Be in conversation with your body. What is your back telling you about this stretch? What are your legs saying? Greet yourself with a face of kindness.

When you are ready to release from the posture, firm your legs, press your feet into the floor, and on an inhalation, lead with your chest to come up to standing. Release your arms back down to your sides, and take a few moments to feel the effects of this posture. What is happening for you now?

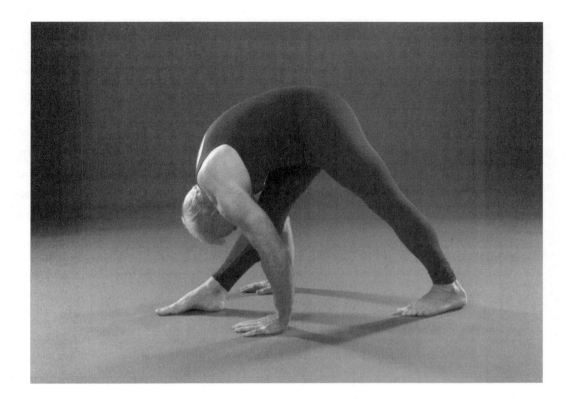

# Standing Forward Bend over One Leg

### Stage One

Begin in Mountain Posture (see Chapter One, Photos 2.1–2.2). Take a few breaths and bring your attention inward. Resolve to stay attuned to the intelligence of your own body.

On an inhalation, jump or walk your feet three and a half to four feet apart. Turn your left leg and foot about seventy degrees to the right. Turn your right leg and foot ninety degrees to the right. Your right heel should be on the same line as the center of your left foot. Place your hands on your hips. Draw your elbows together behind you, and lift your chest.

Turn the front of your trunk from left to right, so that your belly and heart face the same direction as your right foot. Press the outer edge of your left foot firmly into the floor; turn the outside of your left hip forward; straighten and stretch your left leg up and back.

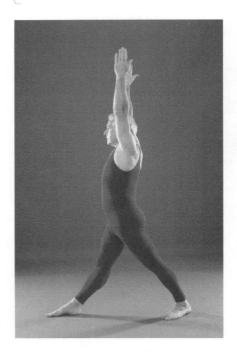

**Photo 24.1**

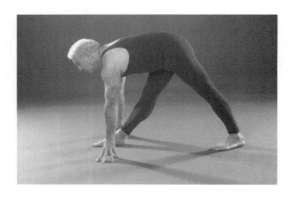

**Photo 24.2**

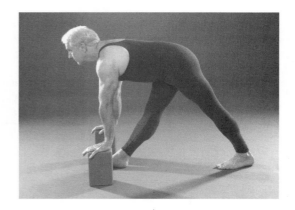

**Photo 24.3**

Press the inner edge of your right foot firmly into the floor, and straighten and stretch the outside of your right hip up and back. Move your tailbone down and in, and check that your pelvis is level.

Extend your two arms out to your sides, palms facing down, and then rotate your arms so that your palms face up. On an inhalation, raise your arms overhead, shoulder-width apart, with the inner creases of your elbows and palms facing each other. Lift both sides of your torso as you lengthen your arms over your head (Photo 24.1).

Draw your tailbone down and in. Inhale and press your back ribs in to lift your chest. Stretch the front of your body up. Take your head back and look up.

On an exhalation, lead with your chest as you bend forward at your hips, extending your trunk and arms forward and down. Bring your fingertips down on the floor, or on blocks on either side of your right foot, and straighten your arms.

Press your feet into the floor and stretch the fronts of your thighs up and back. Lift your kneecaps and lengthen your spine forward. Lift your head and look forward. Move your back ribs in, and lengthen your spine even more, rolling your collarbone and chest up (Photos 24.2–24.3).

Keep weight on your back leg, and continue turning your left thigh and hip to the right. Relax your face and eyes. Give yourself a few moments to arrive fully into this concave part of the posture.

### Stage Two

To go further, bend your elbows out to your sides in order to broaden your chest and draw your torso down over your right leg. Turn your left ribs down, and extend both sides of your torso evenly over your right leg.

Keep stretching both legs up and back. Release the back of your neck, and let your head move toward your shin (Photo 24.4).

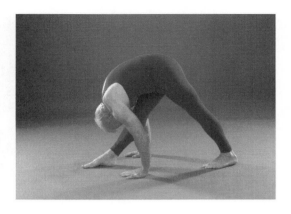

**Photo 24.4**

Move deeper into yourself for three to five breaths. Do not strain to achieve some external goal. The destination of this stretch is you. Quiet your mind; relax your face; be fully present with yourself in this moment of sensation, this moment of you. Trust your intuition to refine your posture.

To come out of the posture, press your left foot firmly into the floor, and on an inhalation, lead with your chest and come to the concave part of the posture for a few breaths.

To come all the way up, on an inhalation, stretch your spine forward and lift your torso upright. Turn your feet to face forward, and jump or step your feet back together. Pause for a moment. Quiet your thoughts and your breath, and be present with yourself in stillness.

Repeat the posture on the other side.

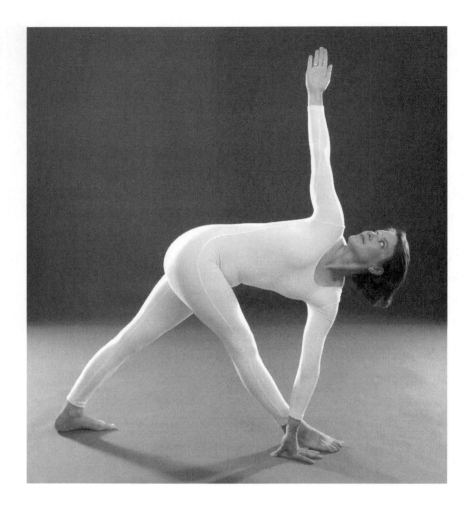

# Revolved Triangle Posture

Join the inner edges of your feet and stand in Mountain Posture (see Chapter One, Photos 2.1–2.2).

On an inhalation, jump or step your feet three and a half to four feet apart. Turn your toes in slightly and your heels out so that the outer edges of your feet run parallel to one another. Stretch your arms out to your sides at shoulder height, and lift and open your chest.

Turn your left leg and foot about seventy degrees to the right. Turn your right leg and foot ninety degrees to the right. Turn your hips and trunk to the right to face the same direction as your right foot. Press your feet firmly into the floor, and stretch your legs up. Lift and open your chest, and stretch your arms sideways.

Press your left heel down, stretch your left leg up, and turn your left outer hip toward the right. Press your right heel and the ball of your big toe down into the floor, and stretch your right thigh up and back (Photo 25.1).

On an exhalation, keeping both legs straight, revolve the front of your trunk from left to right and extend your trunk out over your right leg. Bring your left hand down to the floor on the outside of your right foot. Use a block under your hand if you cannot reach the floor. Place your right hand on your hip. Press both feet firmly into the floor, and stretch both legs up and back.

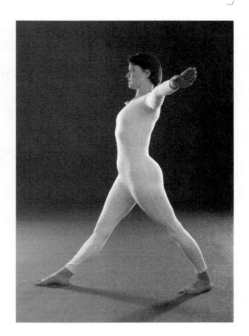

**Photo 25.1**

On an inhalation, lengthen your spine away from your legs and stretch your right arm up toward the ceiling. Stretch your arms away from each other, and press your shoulder blades firmly into your back. Revolve the front of your trunk from left to right while extending your trunk out over your right leg.

Bring the left side of your chest over your right leg, and roll your right shoulder back. Extend both arms away from each other to help you turn more (Photo 25.2).

Finally, turn your head and look up toward your right hand (Photo 25.3).

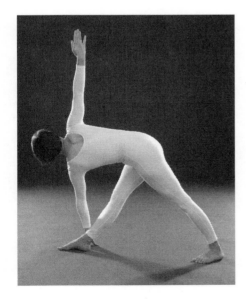

**Photo 25.2**

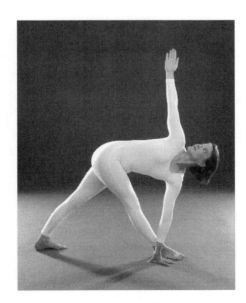

**Photo 25.3**

Breathe evenly as you hold the posture for three to five breaths. This posture has a way of bringing you into intimate and sometimes loud conversation with your whole self.

To release, press both feet firmly into the floor, stretch your legs up, and lift your trunk to stand upright, facing out over your right leg. Then turn your legs and trunk back to center. Rest for a moment.

Repeat the posture to the left.

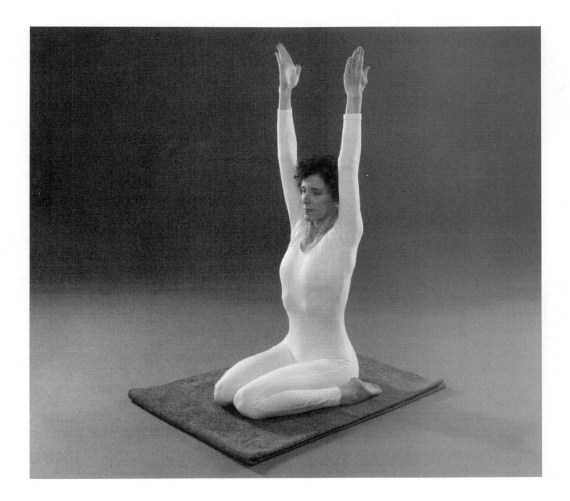

# Hero Posture

Kneel on the floor with your knees and feet hip-width apart, feet and toes pointing straight back.

Bring your knees together and take your feet apart a little wider than your hips. Place your hands in the creases under your knees. Draw your calf muscles toward your heels, and then rotate them outward (Photo 26.1).

As you turn your calf muscles outward, lower your buttocks down and sit between your heels. (Photo 26.2) Quite often, props are necessary in this posture to avoid strain on your knees. If you feel strain, place a firm blanket or block underneath your sitz bones so that your hips are elevated (Photo 26.3).

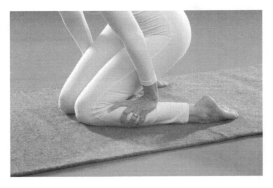

**Photo 26.1**

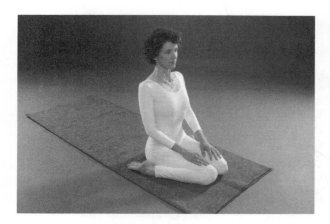

**Photo 26.2**

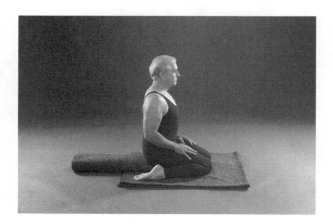

**Photo 26.3**

Pull the flesh of your buttocks out to the sides and diagonally back. Keep your thighs parallel to each other. Stretch your two feet straight back. Rest your hands on your thighs.

Press your buttocks down, and inhale to lift your spine up. Press your shoulder blades into your back to open and lift your chest. Soften your face, your eyes, and the back of your throat.

Extend your arms out sideways, palms facing down. Rotate your arms so that your palms face up. On an inhalation, raise your arms over your head, palms facing each other. Inhale again, and lengthen your arms even more, raising the sides of your torso up off your waist. Keep your tailbone down, lengthen your lower back, and lift and open your chest (Photos 26.4–26.5).

Relax your face and eyes as you hold this posture for three to five breaths. Let your thoughts dissolve into the sensations in your body.

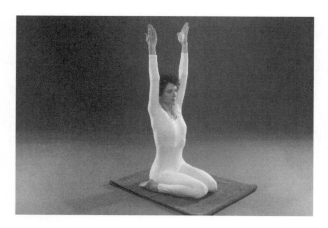

**Photo 26.4**

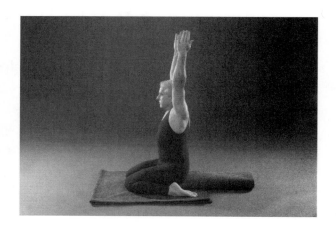

**Photo 26.5**

To release, slowly lower your arms down to your sides. Lean forward and, placing your hands on the floor in front of you, come up onto your hands and knees. Cross your ankles, move your hips back, and sit down in a cross-legged position.

**FREE MOVEMENT**

Take a few minutes now to listen to your body and to move in any way you feel like moving. Quiet any external sources of information, and follow the guidance of your own inner teacher. At first, the voice of your inner teacher may be very quiet, almost imperceptible; in time, it can grow to be very strong and clear. There is no right or wrong way to move freely. Trust your intuition—trust yourself.

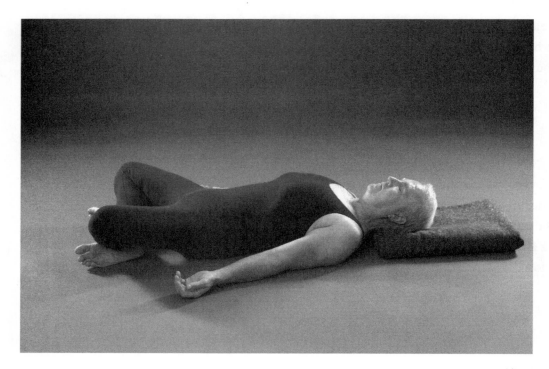

**Photo 27.1**

# Resting Fish Posture

Lie on your back with your knees bent, feet on the floor. Place a firm blanket underneath your head and neck.

Press your feet into the floor to lift your buttocks up slightly, and move your tailbone and buttocks toward your knees. Then lower your buttocks back down.

Cross your legs, and let your knees drop out to the sides. If you feel any strain in your inner thighs, groins, or lower back, place a rolled blanket under each of your thighs.

Relax your arms comfortably down to your sides with your palms facing up (Photo 27.1).

Relax your face. Soften and close your eyes and look inward. Open the door to your inner home, and invite yourself in. Quietly be attentive to yourself as you rest here for a few minutes.

Switch the cross of your legs, and continue resting for a few more minutes. If you notice your mind wandering, gently bring your attention back home to yourself. Observe your breath and your body. Hear your own breath whispering life's secrets.

To come out of the posture, use your hands to draw your knees together. Roll to your right side and rest for a few breaths, curled up in the fetal position. Press your hands into the floor to lift yourself back up to sitting.

# Body Prayer and Alignment
## זוקף כפופים

I N THE EARLY 1800s, in the Polish town of Pshiskha, Rabbi Bunem was asked why he was so late for the morning prayers. He answered: "A person has bones that are still sleeping even after he wakes up." He then explained that because the morning prayers say "All my bones are saying, God, who is like you?" (quoting Psalms 35:10), a person must wait until all his bones wake up before he prays.[1]

Rabbi Bunem did not want to say the prayer "All my bones are saying, God, who is like you?" while his bones were asleep. He wanted his bones themselves to connect with God in prayer, and for that they needed to be awake. Did Rabbi Bunem do something to wake up his bones other than wait? The story does not tell us. However, Sfat Emet teaches that "waking up is making connections."[2] Yoga is a way to actively make connections. With yoga, you can wake up your bones in the morning.

In Jewish tradition, prayer is often called the "service of the heart." Imagine prayer being not only the service of your heart but also the service of your body. Yoga is a way to include the voice of your whole body in your prayers. In so doing, you can align yourself with God and reveal your full essence.

## ⌒ Hearing the Voice of Your Bones

Did your bones wake up when you did this morning, or are they still asleep? Right now, turn your attention inside and sense your bones. Listen to them. What are they saying? Are they singing? Are they praising? Can you remember any time when you felt you were praying with your whole body? Coffee, thank God, is one way to wake up you and your bones; yoga, thank God, can be an even better way!

## Torah Yoga for Body Prayer and Alignment

The prayer called *nishmát kol chai* (the breath of every living thing) says "All my **bones** are saying, 'God who is like you?'" and goes into elaborate detail about how every part of the body is involved in prayer:

> All the **limbs** that You have given us and the **spirit** and **breath** that You have blown into our **noses** and the **tongue** which you have put in our **mouths,** will thank and bless and praise and glorify and sing and exult and adore and make holy and crown Your name, our King, forever. Every **mouth** will thank You and every **tongue** will vow to You and every **eye** will look to You and every **knee** will bend to You and every **straight spine** will bow down in worship before You and every **heart** will be in awe of You and all of the **intestines** and **kidneys** will sing to Your name![3]

Torah, as exemplified in the preceding prayer, teaches that every part of your body can pray. Yoga gives you detailed instruction for waking up every part of your body for prayer.

### Praying with Your Spirit and Body

Rav Kook teaches that although you may not always be conscious of it, your soul is always praying. "The continual prayer of the soul is always striving to come out and reveal itself from its concealed place—to spread out into all the powers of the life of the spirit and into the power of the life of the whole physical body."[4] In other words, your soul's continual prayer wants to make its presence felt and have its voice heard, both in your spirit and in your body. Yoga helps you to feel and hear your soul's continual prayer both spiritually and physically.

### Bent-over and Straight

Rav Kook teaches that a person can be either bent-over or straight, both spiritually and physically.[5] Although you may assume that being bent-over is undesirable, Rav Kook teaches otherwise. Neither posture is appropriate all the time. There are times when being bent-over is appropriate and times when being straight is appropriate. A bent-over, curled-up posture is a way to protect yourself and to gather strength for future tasks. Sleep, for example, is a time of curling up and gathering strength. Sleep is a great and essential blessing.

Nevertheless, in the bent-over posture, your full essence is not revealed. Your essence is revealed when you wake up, uncurl yourself, and lengthen. When you stand straight, you reveal your existential purpose more fully.[6]

Throughout your daily activities—in the work you do, in interacting with others, in praying—stand up to your full height and reveal your full, unique essence. When you stand up tall, you reveal your light. Yoga helps you to "stretch and lengthen all your vital parts and powers, and to reveal them in their full measure"[7]— both to yourself and to the world. Yoga also helps to reveal to you some of the reasons, fears, emotions, and memories that keep you from standing up tall.

## The Blessing of Alignment

There are abundant blessings in the traditional daily Jewish prayer services. Many of them can be experienced in your whole body. As one example of how to pray with your whole body, we will focus on the following blessing from the morning prayers: "Blessed are You, YHVH, our God, King of the Universe, Who straightens the bent-over." This blessing of alignment is an expression of gratitude for being able to stand straight.

With yoga, as your muscles stretch and strengthen and your vertebrae lift up one from the other, you can become a whole-body expression of this daily blessing.

Standing straight is not an isolated act that involves just your spine. Your whole body influences the movement that is possible in your spine. All the postures in yoga can add to the full expression of the blessing of alignment in your body. Imagine yoga postures oiling the squeaky, creaky areas of your body. Imagine drops of lubricating oil between each vertebra of your spine, freeing it up to move, twist, and lengthen gracefully in many directions.

With each posture, you can explore new ways to empower and revitalize your body and spirit. When you lengthen your feet and stretch your toes, you can feel the effect in your spine. As your hamstring muscles become more flexible, your spine can lengthen. Alignment of your pelvis creates an essential foundation for the action in your spine. Back-bends and forward-bends make your spine more flexible. Your breath, bones, muscles—all of you—can participate in the blessing of alignment.

 ## Stretch Your Spine, Reveal Your Spirit

Hasidic thought says that the physical world is like clothing for a spiritual reality. The infinite God is not accessible to human beings in a purely spiritual state. Your body is your spirit in a form that is accessible to you as a human being. Therefore, to engage in the physical is a way for you to access your spirit.

There is more to standing straight than meets the eye. Because your spine is your infinite spirit clothed in nerves, bones, and muscles, every time you straighten and strengthen your spine, you are revealing more of your underlying infinite spirit. Because your spine houses your spirit—and your spirit is a living, dynamic entity—standing straight is a dynamic, ever changing, and challenging endeavor. Because new aspects of the blessing of standing straight can always be discovered, it is meaningful to say the blessing of alignment every day of your life.

Without conscious work in your body-mind, the natural tendency is for your spine to bend over and become more compressed as life progresses. One can see little children sitting easily on the floor, still blessed with the natural alignment of their young spines. Yet it is common to see older people bent-over and rounded in the back. Yoga helps you to consciously counter unconscious nature's way with your spine. You can continue to grow, to lengthen physically and spiritually, as life moves on. The most supple and aligned yogis are the oldest yogis, who have had many years to practice. Through lengthening, twisting, bending, breathing, inverting, and a myriad array of other creative movements for your body, yoga keeps you supple and strong and therefore keeps your spirit radiant.

 ## Torah Study for Body Prayer and Alignment

The blessing of alignment is one of thirteen blessings in the section of morning prayers called **brachót hasháchar** (blessings of the dawn). Originally, these blessings were said in conjunction with different moments of waking up, getting dressed, and getting out of bed in the morning. The Talmud says that when a person gets out of bed and stands up, he or she should say the blessing of alignment.[8] Let us take a closer look at the Hebrew letters and words of this blessing.

### Meaning in the Shapes of the Letters

A student once pointed out to me that the shapes of the Hebrew letters in the words *zokéf kfufím* (straightens the bent-over) actually illustrate the meaning of the words. Figure 1 shows that the letters in *zokéf* (straightens) are formed around a straight central column, like a spine standing upright in a body.

The *fei* at the end of *zokéf* is a special form of *fei* that appears only at the end of a word. At the end of a word, *fei* is long and straight; in the middle of a word (as you will see), *fei* is curled and round.

In contrast, as shown in Figure 2, all but one of the letters in the word *kfufím* (the bent-over) are short and round, like a person curled up.

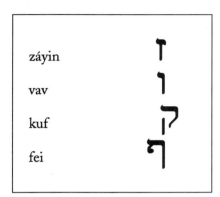

**Figure 1**
*Zokéf* (Straightens)

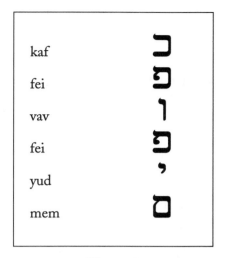

**Figure 2**
*Kfufím* (the Bent-over)

## Connection, Alignment, and Essence

The letter *vav,* which appears in both *zokéf* (straightens) and *kfufím* (the bent-over), is straight up and down. Why is this straight letter in the middle of both words?

The letter *vav* is also the Hebrew word for "and." This letter-word indicates connection between one thing and another. Its shape represents the connection between heaven and earth. When you imitate this letter by standing up straight (as in *zokéf*), you connect and align yourself with heaven and earth. Your powerful essence is expressed by your own personal and unique way of connecting and aligning with heaven and earth. This idea gives meaning to the *vav* in *zokéf* (straightens). Why, though, is there a *vav* in the word *kfufím* (bent-over), when all the other letters are curled up?

According to Rav Kook, even when you are curled up and your essence is not fully revealed, it nevertheless still exists in you in its full character and value.[9] The *vav* found in *kfufím* expresses that, even when you are curled up, you still embody a connection between heaven and earth.

## Aligning with God

The Talmud records a discussion about when to bend over and when to stand straight when saying "Blessed are You, YHVH . . ." at the beginning of the central prayer of the daily services: "Raba bar Chinena [the elder] said in the name of Rav: The one who is praying bends over when saying 'Blessed,' and straightens up when saying YHVH. Shmuel asks what Rav's reasoning is here. Because it is written: YHVH straightens the bent-over."[10] The Talmud instructs us to stand up straight when we refer to God's ineffable name in our prayers. By standing straight while referring to God's ineffable name, we align our mind, body, heart and soul with God and with the full power God has given us.

## The Sound of the Breath and the Shape of the Body

In Jewish tradition, there are many names for God. The ineffable (unutterable) name of God—written in Hebrew with the letters *yud, hei, vav,* and *hei* and transliterated here as YHVH—is found in many blessings. When Jews reading from the Torah or formally praying see the ineffable name of God written, most often they say *adonái* (Lord). Sometimes they say *elohím* (God). These are both Hebrew words and valid names of God, but neither is the actual pronunciation or meaning of YHVH. Any attempt to literally pronounce the ineffable name based on the actual Hebrew letters results in a sound somewhat like breathing.

The four letters of the ineffable name, when written one on top of each other, look somewhat like the shape of the human body (Figure 3). The *yud* is the head. The *hei* is the upper body and arms. The *vav* is the spine. The final *hei* is the pelvis and legs.

When you stand straight, your body resembles the ineffable name of God. When you breathe, you come close to making the sound of the ineffable name of God. In simply standing straight and breathing, you look and sound like the name of God—you exemplify the truth that you are "created in the image of God" (Genesis 1:27).

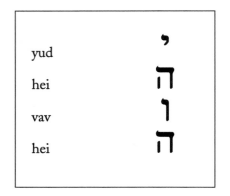

**Figure 3**
YHVH Looking like
a Human Being

## Meaning in the Words

Like most traditional blessings, the blessing of alignment begins with the word *barúch* (blessed). Contained within *barúch* (blessed) is *b'rach* (in softness)—in other words, contained within the blessing is a reminder to be soft. When you practice the daily blessing of alignment, breathe and be soft as you stretch. Do not become rigid in your spine or strained in your body when you align yourself with your powerful essence.

The Talmud teaches that one is obligated to recite at least one hundred blessings a day.[11] All the blessings come to soften the hard places in your life. One hundred times a day, in all the realms of your daily life, bless yourself with the reminder to be soft.

The full beginning phrase of most traditional Jewish blessings is "Blessed are You, YHVH, our God, King of the Universe." Some contemporary Jewish communities have chosen to change the word *king* to *spirit*. One reason for this change is that they object to the patriarchal and authoritarian connotations of *king*. Unfortunately, by changing the word *king* to *spirit*, a beautiful, mystical meaning has been lost. The word **mélech** (king) is made up of the letters **mem, lámed,** and **kaf.** According to Kabbalah, the word **mélech** (king) is an acronym for **móach** (brain—considered the home of the mind), **lev** (heart—considered the home of the emotions), and **klayót** (kidneys—considered the seat of conscience). When invoking the king in the blessings, therefore, one refers not to some storybook image of a powerful male figure on a throne but rather to the very brain, heart, and kidneys of the universe!

A nonliteral translation for the daily blessing of alignment, based on the Hebrew and on Rav Kook's interpretations, is this: Blessed are You, YHVH, brain, heart, and kidneys of the universe, who softly, day by day, straightens us and aligns our essence with You.

When you awake in the morning—and throughout your day—participate fully in the blessing of alignment and stretch to your full height—physically and spiritually.

##  Yoga Practice for Body Prayer and Alignment

Make connections and wake up your bones with yoga. Each posture can be a whole-body expression of the continual prayer of your soul, released and revealed in motion. With each posture, you can actively participate in the blessing of alignment. Alignment is not a rigid holding of your spine and body in one fixed position. You are aligning with your dynamic spirit and with God. Sense the blessing of alignment in your moving spine.

Let yoga help you to become conscious of whatever keeps you from expressing yourself fully. Remember to be soft as you breathe, stretch, lengthen, bend, arch, and twist your way to your powerful essence.

# Meet-Your-Spine Meditation

Bring yourself to a natural standing position. Allow your eyes to soften and close. Invite your attention into your body. Observe yourself without judgment, however you may feel at this moment.

As you stand in this natural position with your focus turning inward, bring your attention to your spine. How is it aligned? Where does it curve? Where is it straight? Where is your head located over your spine? Take a few breaths while you meet your spine in this moment.

Turn your attention to your breath as it comes in and out of your body. Feel each inhalation lift your spine. Gently lengthen and raise your spine, vertebra by vertebra, from your tailbone to the crown of your head. Keep your shoulders rolled back and your chest lifted as you support your lengthening spine with your breath.

Stand straight without being rigid. Relax around your elongating spine. How does this gentle alignment of your spine feel? Is it comfortable or awkward? Does it evoke emotions or memories? Do you feel safe standing this way or vulnerable? Be here, now, fully attentive to your own experience.

Drop your chin toward your chest and allow your shoulders to roll forward, drawing your spine down with them. Bend over, allowing your back and spine to become more rounded. Curl in on yourself. Contract inward. Give yourself your full attention. Does this posture feel familiar or strange? Do you feel comfortable, awkward, scared, or safe?

With your next few breaths, alternate between being *zakúf* (straight) and *kafúf* (bent-over). Inhale as you straighten and exhale as you bend. When you are ready to conclude, come back to a natural standing position. Open your eyes.

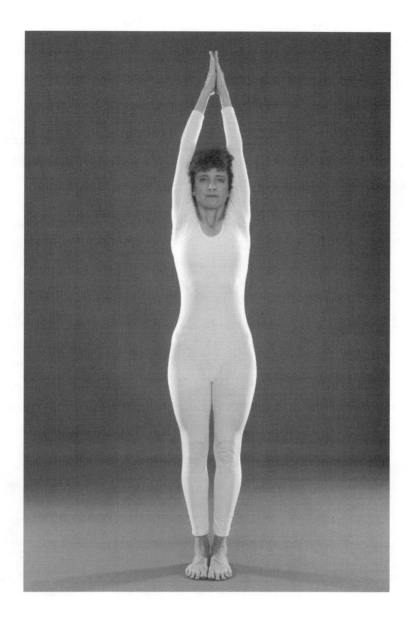

# Upward Reaching Prayer Posture

Begin in Mountain Posture (see Chapter One, Photos 2.1–2.2) with the inner edges of your feet together. Broaden and lengthen your feet as you spread and stretch your toes. Lift the arches of your feet. Press your heels into the floor, and stretch your legs upward. Stretch your arms down by your sides. On an inhalation, lift and lengthen your spine upward. Breathe and be aware.

With each inhalation, lengthen your spine from your tailbone up through the crown of your head. As you lift your spine, roll your shoulders back and down away

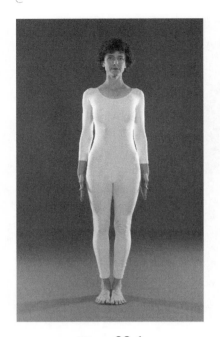

**Photo 28.1**

from your ears. Press your shoulder blades into your back to lift your chest. Relax your belly (Photo 28.1).

On your next inhalation, stretch your arms forward and up, hands shoulder-width apart, palms facing each other. Inhale again, and stretch your arms up toward the ceiling, lifting your ribs and the sides of your torso up from your waist and lengthening through your fingertips (Photos 28.2–28.3).

If possible, keeping your arms straight, bring your palms together and interlace your thumbs. If this is too difficult, keep your arms shoulder-width apart and hold a belt between your hands. Turn your outer arms forward and your inner arms back.

Inhale and stretch your arms even higher. With your head aligned over your spine and your chin parallel to the floor, see that your arms are alongside your ears. Press your shoulder blades into your back and lift your chest more. Keeping your thumbs inter-laced or holding the belt, stretch from the back of your waist up through your fingertips (Photo 28.4).

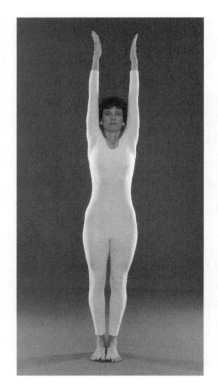

**Photo 28.2**

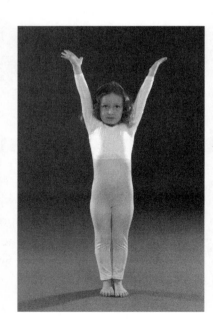

**Photo 28.3**

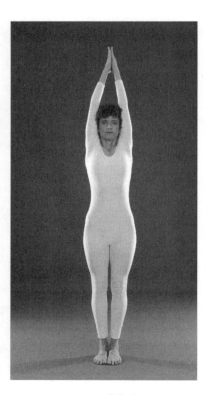

**Photo 28.4**

Hold this posture for three to five breaths, breathing evenly. You are now in the shape of the Hebrew letter *vav*. In this lengthening shape, visualize yourself as the meeting place between heaven and earth. Feel energy flow through you from heaven to earth and from earth to heaven. Breathe into areas that feel tight, closed, or resistant to stretching and lengthening.

To release, lower your arms down to your sides. Pause for a moment and notice how you feel. Repeat the posture, changing the interlacing of your thumbs.

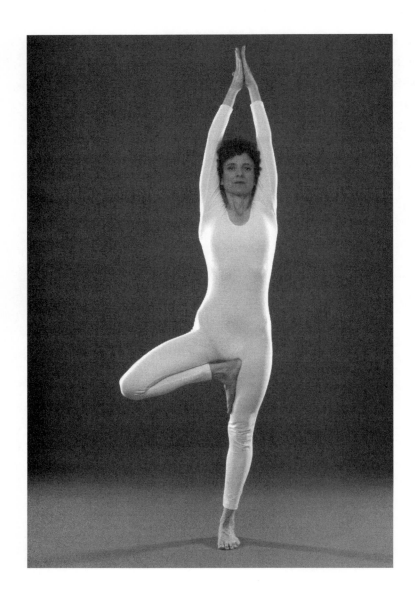

# Tree Posture

Begin in Mountain Posture (see Chapter One, Photos 2.1–2.2). Gather your attention in to your body. Press your feet into the floor, and stretch both legs up firmly.

Press your left heel down and stretch the front of your left thigh up, firming your left knee. Bring your weight onto your left leg as you bend your right knee and turn your right leg out (Photo 29.1).

Keep your eyes relaxed and focused on a point in front of you that is not moving. Raise your right foot and, using your right hand, bring your right heel up into the top of your left inner thigh, toes facing down. Press your right heel into your left inner thigh, and press your left inner thigh back into your right heel.

Turn your right thigh out and back and lengthen it toward the floor as you press your right buttock forward. Stretch from your inner right groin out to your right knee. Firm your left hip as you press your right foot into your left thigh, so that your hip does not jut out to the left (Photo 29.2). Take a few breaths here.

Staying well rooted to the floor, bring your arms out to your sides at shoulder height (Photo 29.3).

Rotate your arms so that your palms face up. On an inhalation, raise your arms up overhead, palms facing each other. On your next inhalation, stretch your arms up further and lift your chest (Photo 29.4). If possible, bring your palms together and interlace your thumbs (Photo 29.5).

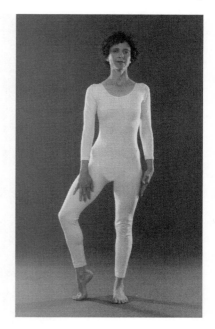

**Photo 29.1**

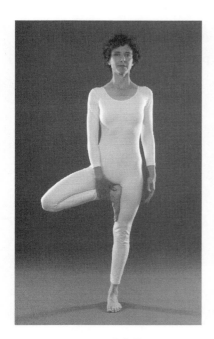

**Photo 29.2**

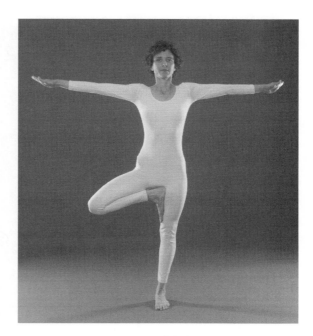

**Photo 29.3**

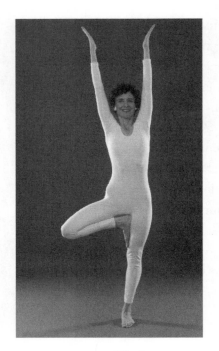

**Photo 29.4**

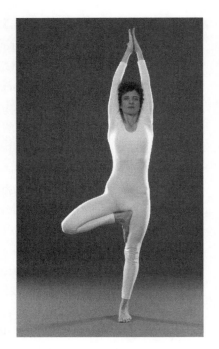

**Photo 29.5**

Balance and grow in this posture for three to five breaths. Soften your breath and relax your face and eyes.

To release, slowly lower your arms and your leg at the same time and come back to standing. Pause and notice how you feel. Repeat on the other side.

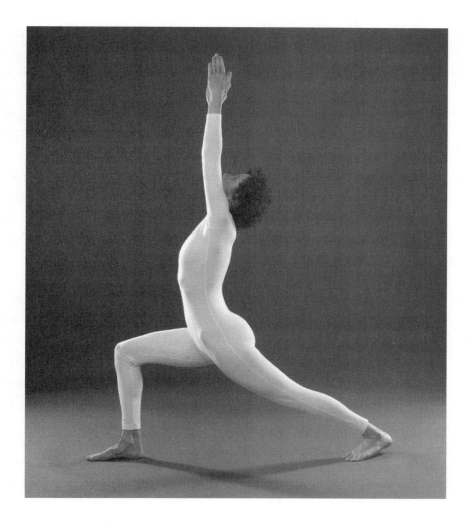

# Warrior One Posture

Begin in Mountain Posture (see Chapter One, Photos 2.1–2.2). Take a few breaths and focus inward.

On an inhalation, step or jump your feet four to four and a half feet apart, stretching your arms out to your sides at shoulder height (Photo 30.1).

Turn your left leg and foot about seventy degrees to the right. Turn your right leg and foot ninety degrees to the right. Line up the heel of your right foot with the heel of your left foot. Inhale and lift and broaden your chest.

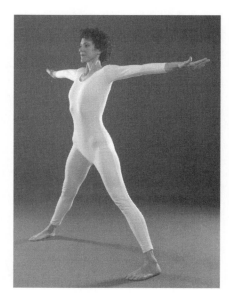

**Photo 30.1**

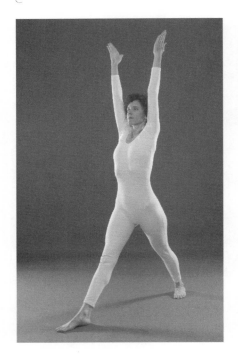

**Photo 30.2**

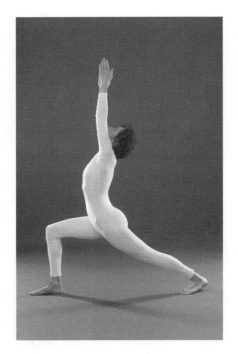

**Photo 30.3**

Turn the front of your trunk from left to right to face the same direction as your right foot. Press the outer edge of your left heel into the floor, and turn your left hip forward. Press your right foot down and stretch your right leg up and back, turning your hips more from left to right. Press both feet into the floor, and stretch both legs up to straighten them.

With your arms stretched out to your sides, rotate your arms so that your palms face up. On an inhalation, raise your arms up overhead, palms facing each other. On your next inhalation, stretch your arms up further and lift your chest. Move your tailbone down and in (Photo 30.2).

On an exhalation, bend your right knee to a ninety-degree angle, bringing your right knee directly over your right heel, right thigh parallel to the floor. (If your knee extends beyond your right heel, adjust the distance between your legs by stepping your left foot back. On the other hand, if your knee is back behind your right heel, step in with your left foot.)

Keeping your right knee bent, press both heels firmly into the floor and stretch and straighten your left leg. On an inhalation, stretch your arms up to lengthen your spine and lift your chest. Press your shoulder blades into your back and downward, expanding your chest even more. Take your head back and look up (Photo 30.3).

Pray here (for strength!) with your whole body for three to five breaths. Relax your breath; soften your eyes and throat; gaze upward with your heart.

To release, press your heels into the floor, inhale, and straighten your right leg. Bring your arms out to your sides at shoulder height. Turn your feet, legs, and trunk to face forward. Walk or jump your feet back together, bringing your arms down to your sides. Soften and observe the effect this posture makes on you.

Repeat the posture on the other side.

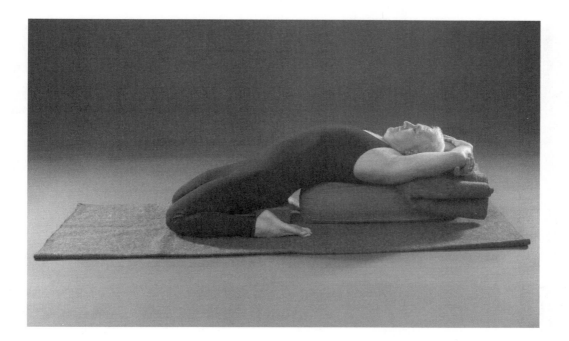

# Reclining Hero Posture

### Option One—With Bolster

Sit in Hero Posture (see Chapter Four, Photos 26.1–26.3), with whatever block or blanket support you might need under your buttocks, if any. Place a bolster lengthwise behind you with a folded blanket at the end of the bolster for your head (Photo 31.1). (If you are already sitting on a support, the bolster should be a few inches higher than the height of your support. If you need more height on your bolster, place a folded blanket lengthwise on your bolster.)

On an exhalation, recline backward, using your hands for support. Lift your buttocks slightly and move your tailbone and buttocks toward your knees; then lower your buttocks back down. Lengthen your spine away from your legs, and lift your chest (Photo 31.2).

Rest the back of your trunk on your bolster with your head and neck supported by your blanket.

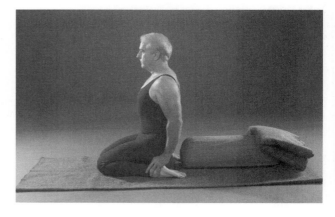

**Photo 31.1**

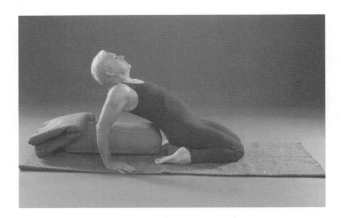

**Photo 31.2**

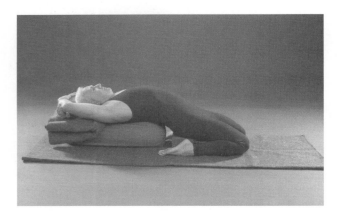

**Photo 31.3**

On an inhalation, stretch your arms over your head, folding your arms and clasping your bent elbows. Stretch the front of your thighs away from your trunk, toward your knees. Press your tailbone into your body, and lengthen your spine away from your legs.

On your inhalations, lift and open your chest. On your exhalations, relax your face and eyes (Photo 31.3).

### Option Two—With Bolster and Chair

If *Option One—With Bolster* is too difficult, try this option. Prop the bolster up against the back of a chair that has been turned upside down and placed against a wall to prevent slipping. Place the bolster on blocks that you can sit on, and place a blanket on top of the bolster for your head (Photo 31.4).

Sit in Hero Posture, and recline backward onto the support of the bolster. Place your hands on your hips (Photo 31.5) or stretch your arms over your head, folding your arms and clasping your bent elbows (Photo 31.6).

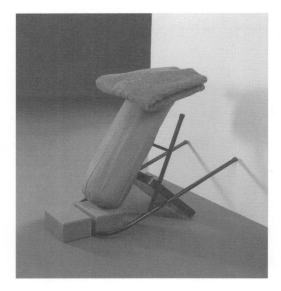

**Photo 31.4**

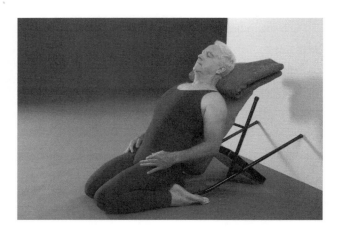

**Photo 31.5**

## Option Three—No Props

You can also practice this posture without props, coming all the way to the floor. When you come to the floor, move your tailbone in and down and stretch your spine away from your legs (Photo 31.7). In this variation, stretch your arms up overhead, palms facing up (Photo 31.8). Although some people lie all the way down on the floor easily, for many it can be quite a challenge for some time. Listen well to your body as you move further into this stretch. Move into this posture, and every posture, as though it were a prayer rather than a competitive gymnastic feat.

Breathe evenly into whatever option for Reclining Hero you practice. Turn your gaze down toward your heart; quiet and relax your busy mind; attend to the world of sensation.

To come out of the posture, bring your hands down by your feet. Press your hands into the floor, and lead with your chest to come back up to Hero Posture. Slowly come up onto your hands and knees. Cross your ankles, move your hips back, and sit down in a cross-legged position.

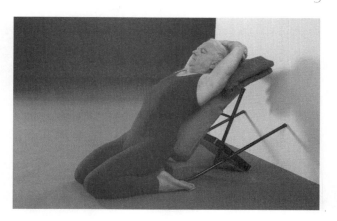

**Photo 31.6**

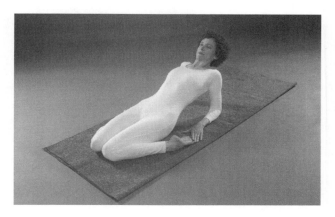

**Photo 31.7**

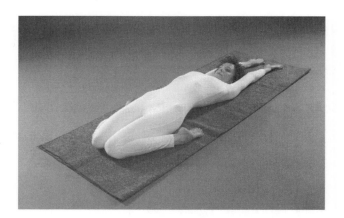

**Photo 31.8**

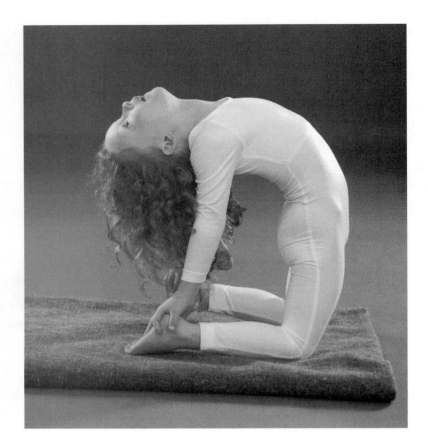

# Camel Posture

Kneel on the floor with your knees and feet hip-width apart, feet and toes pointing straight back.

Press your shins and the tops of your feet firmly into the floor. Press your buttocks forward to bring your hips over your knees, and stretch your thighs upward (Photo 32.1).

Place your hands on your hips. On an inhalation, lift and open your chest. Move your tailbone in as you stretch your spine upward.

On an exhalation, press your back ribs and shoulder blades into your back as you begin to arch backward.

Straighten your arms, and stretch them down and back toward your heels. Bring your hands to your heels, right hand

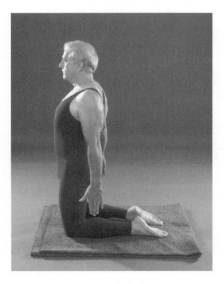

**Photo 32.1**

to your right heel, left hand to your left heel, palms facing down, fingers pointing back. If you cannot get your hands to your heels, place a blanket or bolster over your heels, and stretch your arms back to the blanket or bolster.

Gently release your head back, and lift your back ribs and spine upward. Continue straightening your arms (Photos 32.2–32.3).

With each inhalation, open and broaden your chest. Continue to stretch your legs up and press your buttocks forward, keeping your hips over your knees (Photo 32.4).

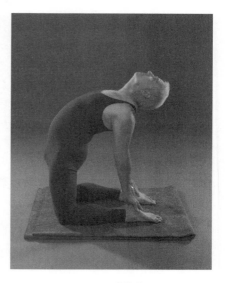

**Photo 32.2**

Stay in this posture for three to five breaths, breathing evenly. Breathe spaciousness into areas that feel tight. Quiet your mind and soften your face. Feel your bones waking up. Listen to your body.

To release from the posture, press your shins and feet into the floor and stretch your legs up even more. Place your hands on your hips and, on an inhalation, lift your chest to come up to a vertical position. Sit back on your feet and observe what happens. Notice how you feel.

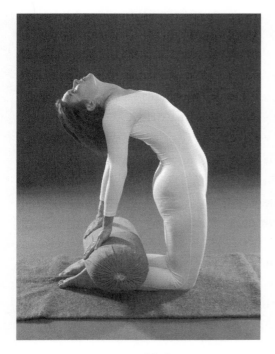

**Photo 32.3**

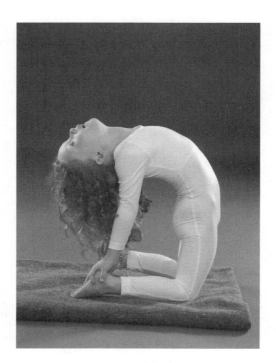

**Photo 32.4**

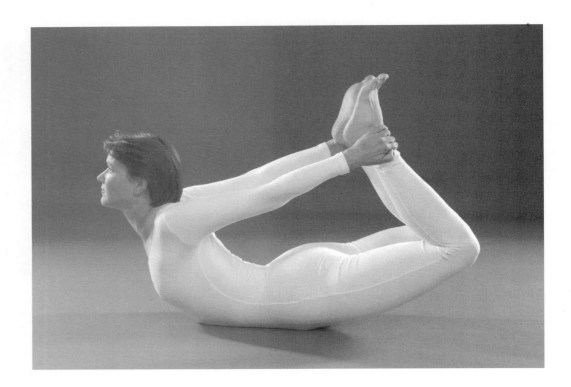

# Bow Posture

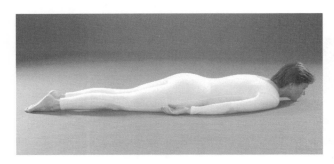

Photo 33.1

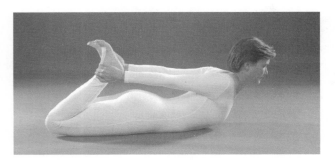

Photo 33.2

Lie on your belly with your arms down by your sides, palms facing up. Rest your chin on the floor (Photo 33.1).

Turn the fronts of your thighs in toward each other, and stretch your legs backward with your knees and feet hip-width apart. Bend your knees, bringing your feet up toward the ceiling. Lift your head and chest off the floor, and stretch your arms back to hold the outside of your ankles with thumbs facing down. If you cannot reach your ankles, use a strap.

Again, turn the fronts of your thighs in toward each other with your knees and feet hip-width apart. Take a few breaths here (Photo 33.2).

On an exhalation, lift your chest higher and pull up on your ankles to lift your knees off the floor. Your arms are now like the taut string of a bow, pulling your legs upward (Photo 33.3).

See that your knees do not go out to the sides. Work at bringing your thighs, ankles, and feet closer together.

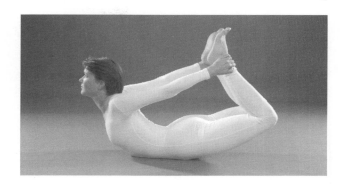

**Photo 33.3**

On your exhalations, lift your chest and arms higher and lift your head as high as possible. Balance your weight on your belly, without hardening your abdominal muscles. The extension and weight on the belly may cause your breath to be short and fast; do not be concerned.

Relax and quiet your breathing as you stay in the posture for three to five breaths. Feel what is happening in your whole body. By now your bones should be very awake!

To come out of the posture, lower your legs and chest to the floor on an exhalation and release the hold on your ankles. Stretch your legs back to rest on the floor.

Repeat the posture two to four times, resting on your belly for several breaths between each bow.

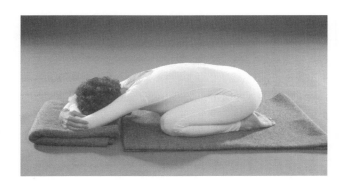

**Photo 33.4**

When you are finished, press your palms down into the floor and come up onto your hands and knees. Move your knees apart, and lower your buttocks to your heels. Relax your trunk forward onto the floor, and rest your forehead on the backs of your forearms on a blanket (Photo 33.4). Alternatively, bring your knees together and rest your arms down by your feet (Photo 33.5)

Rest in this posture for several minutes. Be soft, relaxed, and curled up like the letter *kaf*. This is a posture of resting and gathering strength.

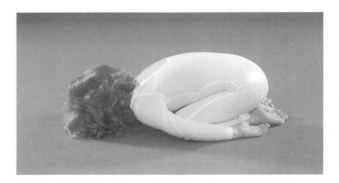

**Photo 33.5**

# Daily Satisfaction

מן לשובע

MANY PEOPLE TODAY feel dissatisfied. In spite of unprecedented material abundance—full fridges and freezers, gizmos and gadgets galore—there are more and more hungry hearts in the big city. Sometimes it seems that our cultural theme song is the Rolling Stones hit "I Can't Get No Satisfaction." Of course, dissatisfaction is not just a modern malady.

In the book of Exodus, the Children of Israel begin complaining just three days after their great deliverance from Egyptian slavery. They complain about not having water. They complain about not having food. Hearing their complaints, God sends them heavenly bread called "manna"—dew-covered honey wafers.[1] During their forty years of desert wandering, manna rains down not only to nourish but also to satisfy the Children of Israel. Moses says to them: "God gives you . . . bread in the morning for satisfaction" (Exodus 16:8).

Heavenly nourishment is still falling. Torah and yoga take you to the fields of your life—places you might even consider desert—to gather there your portion of heavenly bread. With yoga, you can become more aware of the satisfying feast that God showers on you each day. You can learn to trust that every day you receive the divine nourishment you need. You can learn to feel satisfied.

## What Nourishes and Satisfies You?

What heavenly bread is falling onto your plate today? Take a moment to stop and consider: What nourishes your body, mind, heart, and soul? Now go even further. What satisfies you in all these realms? Taste and see the sweet satisfaction of Torah and yoga.

## Torah Yoga for Daily Satisfaction

The parting of the Reed Sea is one of the greatest, most dramatic miracles in the Torah. The sea waters split and stand up like walls so that the Children of Israel can walk safely between them to the other side. Yet even at the height of the miracle, in the middle of the crossing, some can only complain that their shoes are getting muddy![2] If even a biblical miracle is not satisfying, what is?

Ultimately, the outer world is not the most important factor in finding satisfaction. The most important factor is your inner world, where, consciously or not, you choose what to pay attention to. Do you see only the mud as you walk down the corridors of your life, or do you see the miraculous walls of water on either side of you? Do you concentrate on what you do not have, instead of recognizing all that you are blessed with?

When the Children of Israel are wandering in the desert, God gives them manna to take care of both their hunger and their dissatisfaction. God gives everyone exactly what they need each day, no more and no less. You may ask, "What is the nourishing and satisfying manna in my life? Who stocks my local supermarket shelves with fresh heavenly bread? How do I find these dew-covered honey wafers?"

### Torah as Manna

What is the nourishing and satisfying manna in your life? In answering this question, consider: many things in this world can be like manna and can nourish and satisfy you. For example, beauty, love, kindness, and wisdom are like manna. Torah itself is like manna. For thousands of years, Jews have studied Torah for daily nourishment and satisfaction. When Moses is receiving the Torah, Exodus 34:28 tells us he does not eat bread or drink water for forty days. Tradition says that Moses' satisfying nourishment during these forty days, his manna, is the light of the Torah that God gives him.[3]

### Life Energy as Manna

Here is another possibility for you to consider. There is an inner energy flowing within you that nourishes your body, mind, heart, and soul. The Chinese call this inner energy *chi*. Chi reminds me of the Hebrew word *chai* (alive). Let me suggest that the inner energy that flows through you is the energy of life itself. Yogis call the life energy *prana*. *Prana* reminds me of the word manna. For me, my life energy is like manna. Imagine your own life energy as a hearty slice of heavenly bread, with God giving you just the right amount to nourish and satisfy you every day.

Many healing traditions teach that for vitality and good health your life energy must flow freely. Stagnant or blocked energy can lead to distress and even disease. Yoga postures release blocks so that your life energy can flow freely. Yoga teaches you to turn your attention inward and to sense the life energy within you. Sometimes it is subtle like the flutter of a butterfly wing. Sometimes it is powerful like the waves in the ocean. Sometimes it can be sensed as vibration, heat, or color. When you are doing postures, feel the flow of your life energy through your body, mind, heart, and soul.

## God—The Source

Who stocks your local supermarket shelves with fresh heavenly bread? What is the source of your life energy? The Torah teaches that the source is, of course, God. "For with You is the source of Life" (Psalms 36:10). In the story of creating Adam, the Torah says: "And He blows into his nostrils the breath of life" (Genesis 2:7). In the same way that God miraculously rains manna down to feed the Children of Israel, God blows the breath of life right into our nostrils. In other words, God gives us life energy, breath by breath. This is why, in yoga and in all of life, breathing well is such an essential key to keeping your life energy flowing freely.

## A Mystic Dining In—A Satisfying Daily Feast

How do you find your manna, your dew-covered honey wafers? In his popular song "On the Road to Find Out," Cat Stevens suggests that the answers to life's questions lie within. Mystics agree. Mathew Fox, a modern theologian and mystic, defines *mysticism* as turning inward to get your needs met. He opposes this to *addiction*, which he defines as looking outside yourself to get your needs met.[4]

Yoga can teach you to be a mystic, turning inward to get your needs met. With your mystic eyes, you can find manna from heaven within you. You can taste its sweetness in the sensations of your own breath and body. You can gather your daily portion of manna from your own inner supermarket. And it is all organic!

In a recent interview in honor of his eighty-fourth birthday, yoga master B.K.S. Iyengar said of yoga, "Practice is my feast."[5] Yoga is a feast for your body, mind, heart, and soul. It is a feast with many courses and flavors. It is a feast of quiet, a feast of movement, a feast of sensation, a feast of energy, a feast of repose.

An early seventeenth-century Torah commentary teaches that all the different tastes in the world are contained within manna. Because it has all the tastes in the world, everyone can find in manna a taste that he or she likes, everyone can find it satisfying.[6] Likewise, there are many different styles of yoga, each with its unique flavor, so that everyone can do yoga that satisfies. Even within one style, on any given day, you may discover a flavor in your yoga that you never tasted before and that is just what you need.

Like a delicious meal, yoga can be very nourishing and satisfying. It can feel good, pleasurable, and even blissful. Although sometimes it is quite strenuous and difficult, it should not be distasteful or painful. If it is, you need to adjust what you are doing. At your great feast of yoga today, look for and find what you need to be nourished and satisfied.

Physical food, of course, is a necessity that can be nourishing and satisfying. There are, however, many times when nourishment and satisfaction—the tastes you are looking for—are more likely to be obtained from a yoga posture than from the refrigerator.

## The Practice of Satisfaction

Being satisfied is a blessing—a blessing one can practice and learn to feel. There is much to learn about being satisfied from the story of the manna. God gives the Children of Israel a satisfying portion of manna every day. They receive just what they need—no more, no less. They are not supposed to save it for the next day; if they do, it rots. The story of the manna can teach you to trust that today's fresh heavenly bread is satisfying, and that you can receive just what you need.

Just as only today's manna is fresh and satisfying, only today's yoga is fresh and satisfying. When you eat, satisfaction comes from a pleasurable taste in your mouth and the feeling of a comfortably full belly. When you do yoga, satisfaction comes from the joy of liberating and enlivening movements and a sense of nourishing and vital energy flowing through your body. Satisfaction is not in the posture you may be able to do tomorrow or the one you saw someone doing yesterday. Satisfaction is in the stretch you are doing now and in the breath you are breathing now.

## Torah Study for Daily Satisfaction

One morning, early in their desert wanderings, the Children of Israel wake up to find the ground covered with something they have never seen before: dew-covered honey wafers called manna. Moses tells them, "It is the bread that God is giving you to eat" (Exodus 16:15). For forty years, the Children of Israel eat this bread.

What exactly is manna? We know from Moses that it is bread—but we see that it is not ordinary bread. Its miraculous taste and origin, as well as God's commandments concerning it, set manna apart. Yet on consideration, we find that manna teaches that everything ordinary is actually just as miraculous as manna. Moreover, manna teaches how to trust in God and how to find satisfaction.

## Taste of Manna

Manna does not taste like ordinary bread. The Torah says that manna tastes like wafers made with honey (Exodus 16:31). However, as we saw earlier, commentaries say that manna has within itself all the tastes in the world. Because manna has all the tastes in the world, everyone can find it satisfying. Although manna itself is clearly miraculous, it is perhaps no more miraculous than the world itself. The world also contains all tastes within it, and potentially everyone can find it satisfying too.

## Origin of Manna

The process of preparing ordinary bread for eating is quite complicated. People must plant grain at the proper times and places. The grain requires the proper amounts of sun and water in order to grow. Then, God willing, the grain grows. Finally, people must harvest the grain, grind it into flour, and bake it into bread.

The process of preparing manna for eating is much less complicated. Manna falls from heaven at the times and places that God commands. God says, "Here I am, raining down for you bread from heaven" (Exodus 16:4). People must still go out and gather the manna at the proper times.

Although there are clearly differences in these details, in essence, the origins of ordinary bread and manna are the same. Specifically, both require God and people working together to obtain the desired result: nourishment and satisfaction.

In the traditional Jewish blessing for bread, we do not acknowledge the human hand in the bread-making process. We skip right to the divine source: "Blessed are You, YHVH, our God, King of the Universe, *who brings bread out of the earth.*"[7] In the same way that God brings bread from the earth, God rains manna from heaven. Thus, in the traditional view, there is no such thing as ordinary bread—ordinary bread is as miraculous and divine as manna. In fact, in the traditional view, ultimately, all food comes from God.

## God's Commandments

Moses tells the Children of Israel about God's commandments regarding the manna. They are commanded to gather the manna "according to what they need—one *ómer* [less than two quarts][8] of manna, per person, per day" (Exodus 16:16). There seems to be a contradiction here. How can it be that people's differing needs always turn out to be a standardized portion—one *ómer* per person per day? The commentaries explain that it is a miracle that one *ómer* of heavenly bread per person per day *satisfies* everybody—whether they are used to eating a little or a lot.[9]

When the Children of Israel actually do go out to gather manna, some gather a little and some gather a lot. When they come back from the fields and measure how much they have gathered, another miracle occurs. It turns out that they always end up with exactly one *ómer* of manna per person—no more and no less![10] The exception to this one-*ómer* rule is on Friday. Every Friday they end up with double the usual amount. Moses explains that because manna does not fall on Shabbat (Friday night to Saturday night), God doubles the amount of manna on Friday (Exodus 16:22, 23). According to God's commandment, Friday is the only day they can save some manna for the next day. The rest of the week, if they try to save manna for another day, it gets wormy and rots.

What do God's commandments concerning manna teach us?

## Trusting God's Providence

At first, the Children of Israel try to do it their own way. Some gather a little, some gather a lot, but nevertheless everyone ends up with one *ómer* per person per day. Some try to save up manna and hoard it for subsequent days, but it rots. Some go out to gather it on Shabbat but find none. Try as they may, they only get exactly what they need for each day.

For forty years, God sends the manna, with all its miraculous ways, to teach the Children of Israel to trust that day by day God provides just what they need. With manna as their food, they have no choice but to trust in God's providence. It takes time for the Children of Israel to learn this lesson. It is a lesson we are still learning today.

## Eating Manna—Knowing God

Manna and God are inextricable. Eating manna connects you to God. Actually, eating manna is a way to know God. The first passage about manna says, "In the morning you will be satisfied with bread, and you will know that I am YHVH, your God" (Exodus 16:12). Later the Torah says: "And He gives you manna to eat . . . in order to teach you that man does not live by bread alone—man lives by anything that comes from the mouth of God" (Deuteronomy 8:3).

When Moses is up on the mountain receiving the Torah, he does not eat bread or drink water for forty days. What does he eat? How does he live? A thirteenth-century commentator and Kabbalist, Rabbeinu Bachya, says that Moses receives nourishment from the highest light. He also says that in the world to come the righteous live and are nourished by the quality of loving-kindness and from the radiance of the highest light.[11] Rabbeinu Bachya calls spiritual food the true nourishment. The psalmist says: "Taste, and see that God is good" (Psalms 34:9).

## Gather from God

In the first instruction about the manna, there is a hint that the nourishment the Children of Israel are supposed to gather from the fields is spiritual nourishment. "Every person should gather *from it* according to his needs" (Exodus 16:16). Why does this passage say that each person should gather "from it" and not gather "from the manna"? "From it" in this passage is the translation of the word *miménu.* This word also means "from Him," referring to God. In other words, go out and gather from God. Gather from God's energy, gather from God's goodness, and gather from God's light. Whether we are up on the mountain with Moses or in the fields gathering bread, there is soul food from God that we can gather. When you gather from God, you are assured to get the perfect measure and taste that you need.

## Satisfaction

The Torah mentions several times that manna is satisfying bread. What is it about manna that makes it satisfying? Perhaps it is because of its inextricable connection with God. Bread alone is not satisfying. Bread with God is satisfying.

The blessing after food says, "God nourishes the whole world with His Goodness."[12] In the Shabbat prayers, we say to God, "satisfy us with Your Goodness."[13] Perhaps satisfaction comes with your daily portion of true nourishment, God's goodness.

At the end of the story of the manna, God tells Moses to save a jarful of manna to remind people throughout the generations that God continues to provide nourishment and satisfaction for the world (Exodus 16:33). Three times a day in the traditional prayers, we say: "God opens His hand and satisfies all that live."[14]

Discover the miracles of manna everywhere. Taste it in your bread. Feel it in your movements. Sense it in your breath. May we all be blessed to gather satisfying heavenly bread from all the many fields of life.

 ## Yoga Practice for Daily Satisfaction

The mystic turns inward for his divine feast. Let your eyes, which so often look outward, relax. Open up your inner eyes. Go to your inner fields and gather your manna.

In each posture, feel the nourishing sensations and energy of your moving breath and body. Taste the heavenly bread of satisfaction in each stage of every posture while you are doing it. What you need today is falling like manna in just the right measure.

# Centering Meditation

Sit on a firm folded blanket with your buttocks on the blanket and your feet on the floor. Cross your legs. Soften your upper groins, and release the tops of your thighs down toward the floor (see Chapter One, Photo 1.1).

Root yourself down through your sitz bones and inhale to lengthen your spine upward. Draw your shoulder blades into your back, and expand and lift your chest. Lift your head upward, with your chin parallel to the floor. Rest your hands on your knees, palms facing up, fingers relaxed.

Gaze inward. Close your eyelids gently. This is the time to be a mystic and gather manna from within.

Feel your breath. Listen to your breath. Ponder on the mystery of where your breath originates. Sense the subtle ways your breath is giving every cell in your body just what it needs in just the right measure. Feel how much satisfaction there is in breathing.

Now take a few deep, slow breaths into your whole body. Notice in your body an inner nourishing field of divine energy. Affirm that what you need to be satisfied today is within you.

Knowing that you are going to deepen your connection to the manna within you in your yoga practice, open your eyes.

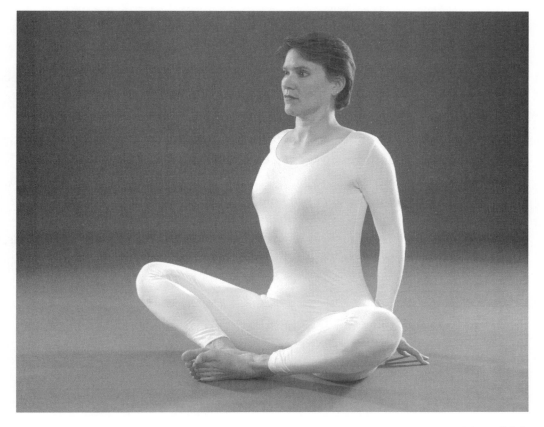

**Photo 34.1**

# Cobbler Posture

Sit on the floor in Staff Posture (see Chapter Three, Photo 15.1).

Turn your legs out slightly and bend both knees. Bring the soles of your feet together, and extend your knees out to the sides.

Pull your feet in close to you, and press your heels firmly together.

If your knees are higher than your pelvic bones, sit up on a blanket or two so that you can lower your knees below the level of the top of your pelvis.

Bring your hands back by the sides of your hips. Press your fingertips into the floor or blanket, and lift and lengthen your spine upward. Press your shoulder blades into your back. Turn the tips of your elbows back, and roll the outer corners of your shoulders back. Open and broaden your chest.

Pressing your feet together, extend your inner thighs from groin to knee and lower your knees down toward the floor.

Draw your outer thighs from your outer knees back toward your buttocks. Press your buttocks firmly into the back of your pelvis.

Keep your buttocks on the blanket as you lift and lengthen your spine, and broaden your thighs away from each other (Photo 34.1).

Relax your breath as you hold this position for five to ten breaths.

To release, bring your hands to your outer knees and, using your hands, bring your knees together. Then straighten your legs.

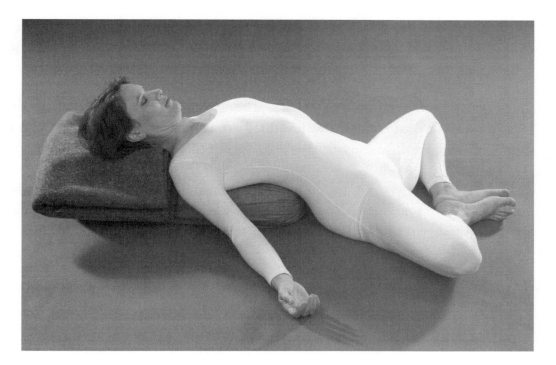

**Photo 35.1**

# Supported Cobbler Posture

Sit on the floor, and place a bolster lengthwise behind your buttocks with a folded blanket at the end of the bolster for your head.

Bring the soles of your feet together and draw them in close to you, as in Cobbler Posture (see this chapter, Photo 34.1).

On an exhalation, and using your hands for support, rest the back of your trunk on your bolster, with your spine along the center of the bolster and your head and neck supported by your blanket. After lying down, lift your buttocks slightly and move your tailbone and buttocks toward your knees, then lower your buttocks back down. Lift your chest, and draw your shoulder blades in and down toward your waist.

Release your thighs from your inner groin to your knee. If you feel strain in your thighs, groin, or lower back, place a rolled blanket underneath your thighs and calves for support.

Move your tailbone in and down again. Open your heart. Feel the support of the bolster and relax. Stretch your arms out to your sides, palms facing up (Photo 35.1).

Soften and close your eyes, and bring your attention inside. Release into this supported stretch. Be here breathing evenly for a few minutes. Quiet your mind, and open up to the satisfying sensations of this stretch.

To come out of the posture, use your hands to draw your knees together. Roll to your right side and rest for a few breaths, curled up in the fetal position. Press your hands into the floor to lift yourself back up to sitting.

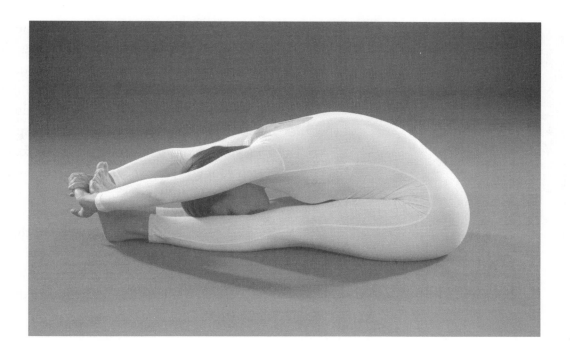

# Sitting Forward Bend

### Stage One

Sit with your legs extended out in front of you in Staff Posture (see Chapter Three, Photo 15.1). If your lower back rounds, sit on the edge of a firm folded blanket. Pull the flesh of your buttocks out and diagonally back, and sit evenly on your sitz bones. Press out through your heels and the balls of your feet.

Place your hands down at the sides of your hips with your fingers facing forward. Press your hands into the floor or blanket, and lengthen your spine upward. Roll your upper thighs in toward each other, press your thighs toward the floor, and inhale to lengthen your spine up more, lifting and expanding your chest (Photo 36.1).

Continue to press your legs down toward the floor, and lift your chest as you extend your torso and spine up and over your legs. Stretch your arms forward, and hold the sides of your feet with your hands; alternatively, wrap a belt under the balls of your feet, and hold the sides of the belt.

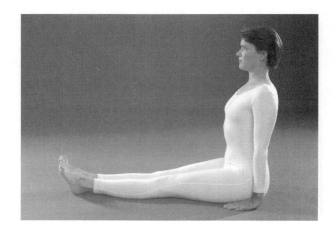

**Photo 36.1**

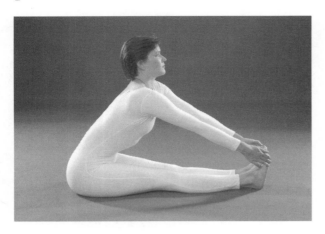

**Photo 36.2**

Straighten your arms, and turn the inner creases of your arms up to face the ceiling. Pull with your arms to move your back ribs in, lift your chest, and roll your collarbone up toward the ceiling. Press your upper thighs toward the floor and inhale as you lengthen the front of your spine from your pubis up to your chest. Look forward; soften your eyes; breathe into places that are tight or resistant (Photo 36.2).

Feel yourself in this concave part of the posture for a few breaths. Do not race ahead to the next part. Every stage of the posture has a taste; every stretch is nourishing; every breath distributes energy.

## Stage Two

When you are ready, breath by breath, move deeper into the posture. Continually press your upper thighs into the floor. Inhale to lengthen your spine. Exhale to extend forward over your legs, bending from your hips. Bend your elbows, lift them up and out to your sides, and lengthen the front of your ribs and spine up and over your legs. Rest your forehead down on your shins or on a blanket or bolster placed on top of your legs (Photos 36.3 and 36.4).

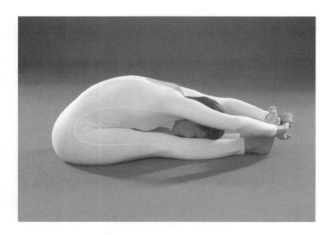

**Photo 36.3**

Optionally, if you are well extended over your legs, you can switch your hand position. Turn your palms to face away from you. Hold the back of your right hand or wrist with your left hand, and place the backs of your hands on the balls of your feet. Press your hands into your feet to lengthen your spine over your legs.

Hold this position for five to seven breaths. Each time you come to a new limit, let your thoughts be absorbed in the sensations in your body. Release any preoccupation with how far you can bend. Forward bends provide an excellent opportunity to practice being present and patient at each stage of the posture. Feast on each breath. Feel the effects of each subtle adjustment.

To release, press firmly into your legs and come back to the concave part of the posture. Place your hands on the floor on the sides of your hips and inhale, as you return to your upright position.

Take a moment to soften and absorb the nourishing benefits of this stretch. Affirm that you are satisfied with what you have done.

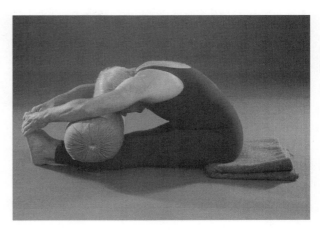

**Photo 36.4**

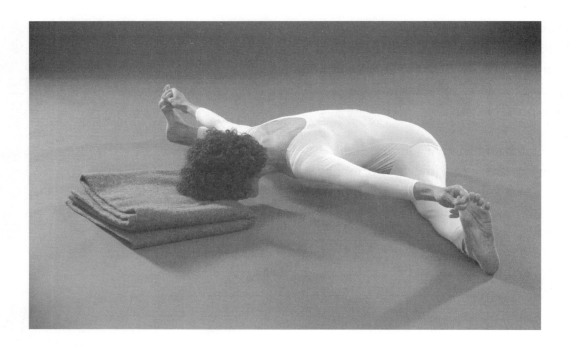

# Seated Angle Posture

## Stage One—Upright

Sit on the floor in Staff Posture (see Chapter Three, Photo 15.1). One leg at a time, take your legs wide apart. See that the tops of your thighs, knees, shins, ankles, and toes face straight up toward the ceiling.

If your lower back rounds out when sitting on the floor, sit on a folded blanket or two so that you can straighten it.

Bring your hands back by the sides of your hips, press your fingertips into the floor, and lift and lengthen your spine upward. Press your shoulder blades into your back, and lift your chest. Bend your elbows slightly, turn the tips of your elbows back, and roll the outer corners of your shoulders back. Open and broaden your chest.

Press your thighs and shins down toward the floor, and lengthen the backs of your legs out toward your heels.

Draw your outer thighs from your outer knees back toward your buttocks. Press your buttocks firmly into the back of your pelvis (Photo 37.1).

Hold this position for three to five breaths. Relax your breath.

### Stage Two—Twisting

On an exhalation, turn the front of your trunk from left to right. Bring your left hand to the floor between your legs, and bring your right hand back behind your left buttock.

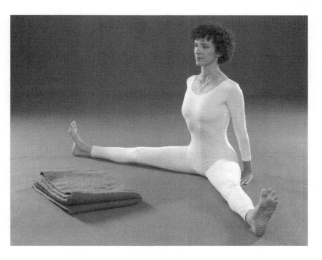

**Photo 37.1**

Press your left buttock down, and extend your left leg out to the left. Roll your outer left thigh down to prevent your left leg from turning in too much.

Press your fingertips down into the floor, and lift your spine up. Use your breath to help you turn from left to right: on your inhalations, lift and extend your spine upward; on your exhalations, turn your trunk from left to right.

Roll both outer shoulders back. Draw your shoulder blades into your back, and broaden your chest as you turn (Photo 37.2).

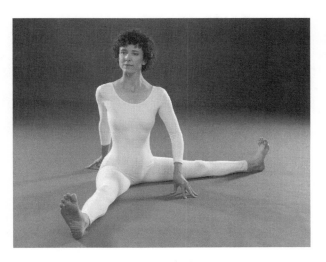

**Photo 37.2**

Stay in this position for five to seven breaths. Keep your inner eyes open and watchful for manna each time you turn.

On an exhalation, return to center; then repeat to the left.

### Stage Three—Forward Bend

From the upright position facing forward, stretch your torso forward slightly and reach out sideways with your arms and hands toward each foot. If you can, make a ring grip around your big toes—right thumb, index, and middle fingers around your right big toe; left thumb, index, and middle fingers around your left big toe. If you cannot reach your big toes, hold your ankles, or use straps around the soles of your feet.

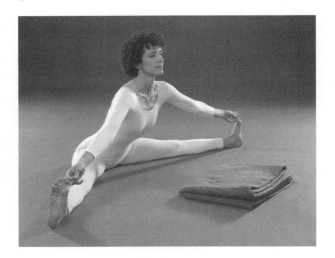

**Photo 37.3**

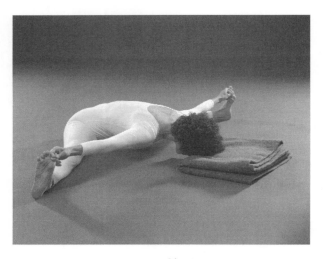

**Photo 37.4**

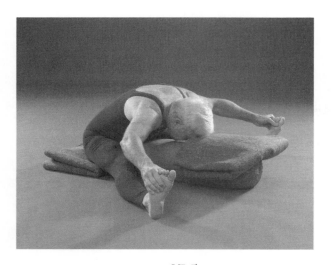

**Photo 37.5**

Pull on your big toes, stretch your arms, and make your back concave by lifting your chest and diaphragm upward. Press out through the balls of your feet, and move your thighbones down toward the floor (Photo 37.3).

Stay in this concave position for two to four breaths, breathing evenly. Deeply involve yourself in each stage of the posture. Let go of the tendency to anticipate what is coming next rather than experiencing what is happening now.

On an exhalation, extend your trunk forward, and rest your forehead on the floor in front of you (Photo 37.4). If you cannot get your head to the floor, place a blanket or bolster in front of you, and lower your head and trunk to that height. (Photo 37.5). Inhale and lengthen your spine. Exhale and extend your spine forward, taking your back ribs in and extending the front of your trunk forward. Broaden your chest from the middle of your chest out to the sides.

Press your outer thighs down to prevent your legs from turning in, and move your buttocks down toward the floor. You can even use your hands to roll your outer thighs down (Photo 37.6).

When you come to a place of tension, breathe, wait, and notice. Be patient and attentive as sensations intensify, and then relax. Move as though you were taking small bites of delicious food. Savor each bite as you chew it.

Stay in this forward extension for three to five breaths. Relax your breath. Soften the skin on your face, your eyes, and the back of your throat.

On an inhalation, come back to the concave position, holding your big toes. Lift your chest and extend your spine up.

Release the hold on your big toes, inhale again, and come to the upright position. Then bring your legs together and relax. Pause a moment to taste the benefits of the posture you have just done.

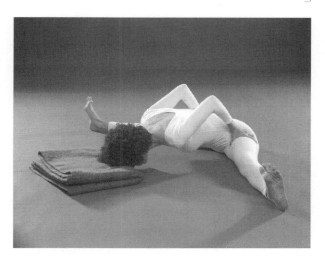

**Photo 37.6**

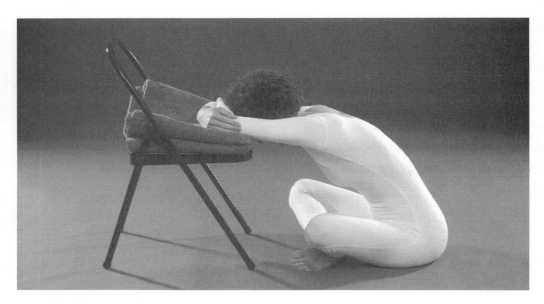

**Photo 38.1**

# Supported Cross-Legged Forward Bend

Sit cross-legged in front of the seat of a chair. If your lower back rounds, sit on a folded blanket with your feet on the floor. If the seat of the chair is hard, place a folded blanket on it.

Raise your arms up overhead and fold your arms, holding your elbows. Keeping your tailbone down, bend forward. Rest your forehead on the edge of the chair; rest your folded arms up on the chair seat (Photo 38.1).

Adjust the chair to whatever distance gives you the stretch in your spine that you want. You do not have to stretch to your full extension. Soften and close your eyes, and let your brain relax. Draw your senses of perception inward. Sense the subtle vibrations of nourishing energy moving through your body. Notice how satisfying it can be to stretch gently, breathe, and relax. Spend a few minutes here, and enjoy the fine delicacy of rest and repose.

To release, inhale and come up to an upright sitting position. Change the cross of your legs and the fold of your arms, and repeat the posture.

# Remembering to Rest

## שבת מנוחה

**M**ANY PEOPLE FEEL that they cannot take the time to rest. They are too busy. They think that, at least while they have the strength, resting is something they can always do later. It often seems that they frown on resting and consider it a waste of time or a frivolous indulgence.

Torah has a radically different attitude toward resting. In the Torah, the fourth of the Ten Commandments commands us to always remember and observe Shabbat (Friday night to Saturday night). Shabbat is a day for soulful, holy rest. The day of rest is adored and desired like a beloved soul mate. It is a bride and queen, the crown of every week. Shabbat teaches us how to rest.

Yoga also teaches us how to rest. In yoga, rest and relaxation are an essential part of the practice. The climax of every yoga session is the posture of rest.

Jewish tradition teaches that God's ability to stop working and rest on Shabbat is an example of immense strength.[1] It takes strength to stop and rest. Both Shabbat and yoga can help you to be strong enough to stop working. They can teach you the art of resting.

##  Is It Time to Rest Yet?

Take a deep breath right now, and then let it go. Consider: How busy are you? What is your attitude about resting? Do you ever allow yourself to stop and rest in the middle of your work? There is a time to work and a time to rest. Keep the rhythm of your life soulful—remember to rest.

## Torah Yoga for Remembering to Rest

I remember the day that I decided to be less busy in my life. After several years of observing Shabbat and practicing yoga, I began to sense a rhythm different from the one around me—a slower, quieter, more soulful rhythm. I decided to leave my very busy teaching job where we were teaching children to be very busy.

At that time, people would often ask me: "Are you keeping busy?" There was an unspoken implication in the tone of the question that somehow I should be busy, that if I was busy I was doing something right. It seemed that there was something threatening to people about my not being busy. What I really wanted to answer was "No, I am not busy, thank God." I was beginning to sense that God had something to do with not being busy.

### Remember to Take a Deep Breath

When the Jewish people were slaves in Egypt, they were very busy. They worked every day. They were so lost in their hard work that, for a long time, they did not even stop to take a deep breath. One day, something changed within them, and they sighed. God heard their sighs, took them out of slavery (Exodus 2:23 ff.), and gave them Shabbat (in the Torah), the great gift of rest. God commanded them to remember and observe Shabbat (Exodus 20:8; Deuteronomy 5:12), to ensure that they would never become slaves to their work again.

Both Shabbat and yoga remind you to free yourself from your busy life, to take a deep breath, and to make time for resting. If you wait until all your work is done before resting, you will never get to rest. If you wait until you have time before doing yoga, you will never do it. Resting is a conscious choice to shift your attention from the busy activities of your life to something else. You may need to leave your e-mails unanswered in order to light your Shabbat candles. You may need to leave dishes in the sink in order to get to a yoga class. You can almost count on it: Shabbat and your yoga classes will come right in the middle of very important work that you feel you must do. The truth is that resting also means leaving something unfinished. Remember, however, that you are in good company. According to Jewish tradition, God stopped working and rested on Shabbat even though the world itself was not completely finished.[2] The concept of *tikún olám* (fixing the world) teaches that we humans are partners with God in completing the work of creation.

## Restorative Postures

Within you, at the root of your being, there is a place of rest. The Hebrew word *tnuchá* (posture) is built from the root word *nóach* (rest). Resting and relaxation are at the root of yoga postures. Yoga postures take you inside to the root of rest within yourself where you can experience resting in the cells of your body.

Yoga postures can be divided into different categories. There are restorative postures that are usually effortless and relaxing. There are standing postures, back-bends, forward-bends, twists, and inversions that often require a lot of effort. Ultimately though, all yoga postures can and should be done in a relaxed, effort-less way. It takes practice, however, to learn to do this. The sage Patanjali said: "Perfection in a posture is achieved when the effort to perform it becomes effort-less, and the infinite being within is reached."[3]

Practicing restorative postures helps you to experience a deeply restful, even blissful, state of being. Learning to rest and relax in restorative postures makes it easier to bring the restful state into the more active, challenging postures. Learning to be relaxed in the challenging postures is like bringing the peace and rest of Shabbat with you into your workweek.

## The Day of Rest, the Posture of Rest

*Shabbat* is the Hebrew name for the day of rest, the Sabbath, at the end of every week. *Shavasana* is the Sanskrit name for the posture of rest, the Relaxation Posture, practiced at the end of every yoga session. Although they have different literal meanings, they have similar sounds: *shaa–aaah*, like the sounds a mother makes in the middle of the night to soothe her troubled child. Shabbat and yoga are both essentially restful practices that quietly soothe us. Both can help teach us to rest and be relaxed even during the more challenging days and postures of our lives.

##  Torah Study for Remembering to Rest

Recognizing that people do not always make time to rest in their busy lives, traditional Judaism does not leave it to whim or chance. In the Torah, resting on Shabbat is more than a good idea or a friendly suggestion—it is a commandment from God: "Do not do any work, you and your sons and your daughters and your servants and your animals and the stranger who is in your gates" (Exodus 20:10). Not only is resting not a waste of time, or indulgent, it is holy. "God blesses the seventh day and makes it holy because on it He rests from all of His work" (Genesis 2:3). This is the first time the word *holy* is used in the Torah. In a world that worships and glorifies work, Shabbat teaches us the blessed sanctity of rest.

## A Day to Restore Your Soul

The following Torah verse illuminates for us the inseparable connection between Shabbat, resting, and the soul. "In six days God makes heaven and earth, and on the seventh day He stops working and *yinafásh*" (Exodus 31:17). The reflexive Hebrew verb *yinafásh* comes from the same root as *néfesh*. The word *néfesh* is one of five Hebrew words meaning "soul." It also means "rest" and "recuperate." According to the Brown, Driver, and Briggs *Hebrew and English Lexicon of the Old Testament*, one meaning of the verb *yinafásh* is "take breath, refresh oneself."[4] A nineteenth-century Torah commentary teaches that *yinafásh* refers to "the rest and relaxation that restores the soul."[5]

Because the verb *yinafásh* is layered with meaning, there are many ways to understand the Torah verse at Exodus 31:17. Everett Fox, a modern Biblical scholar, translates it as "On the seventh day He ceased and paused for breath."[6] It can also be translated as "On the seventh day He stops working, and rests and restores His soul."

There are teachings that Shabbat is the day that we actually receive our soul. An eighteenth-century Torah commentary teaches that, before the first Shabbat, there was no soul in creation. On Shabbat, God gives us the abundant, essential vitality that *is* our soul.[7] Another opinion is that we receive an extra soul on Shabbat. The Talmudic sage, Resh Lakish, teaches, "On Friday evenings God gives an extra soul to man."[8]

Another one of the five Hebrew words for soul, *n'shamá,* shares the same root as the Hebrew word for breath, *n'shimá.* Just as Hebrew illuminates the connection between resting and your soul, Hebrew illuminates the mysterious unity of your breath and your soul. On Friday evenings, God gives us more breath—more soul.

On Shabbat, we imitate God. Each week when we stop working and rest, when we take a breather, we restore—perhaps even receive—our souls.

## Speaking About the Soul

I do not recall anyone ever talking about the soul when I was growing up. I do not think it was ever mentioned in my public school or even in my Hebrew school. I remember how thrilled I was when, in college, I found a friend with whom I could talk openly about my soul. One of the great poetic and mystic scholars of our century, Rabbi Abraham Joshua Heschel, says that ultimate questions about the soul are the object of man's favorite unawareness. He says: "our theories will go awry, will all throw dust into our eyes, unless we dare to confront not only the world, but the soul as well."[9]

For Rav Kook, on the other hand, the soul seems to be a favorite object of awareness. Hear his words: "My soul sails and flies above everything that can be called by any name. . . . It speaks without logic, it acts without action."[10] When you stop to take a breath—when you rest—your soul can become your favorite object of awareness as well.

Shabbat prayers call Shabbat "the most desired, lovely, delightful day."[11] They call Shabbat resting "a rest of love and generosity, a rest of truth and faith, a rest of peace, serenity, quiet and security, a complete rest."[12] What is the way to this most desirable rest? Let us look at both legal and mystical routes to resting.

## Legal Resting

Resting does not mean just refraining from work. The Torah teaches that resting requires consciously not doing some things and doing other things instead. The fourth commandment says: "Do not do any work on Shabbat" (Exodus 20:10). It also says, "Remember/Observe Shabbat" (Exodus 20:8; Deuteronomy 5:12). Traditional Jewish law, *halachá* (the way), defines exactly what work is—exactly what you may not do on Shabbat. It also defines what you must do in order to remember and observe Shabbat, the divine example of resting.

Jewish tradition forbids many activities of daily living on Shabbat because they are considered work. Driving a car, talking on the phone, and turning on lights are a few examples. Even if you agree that resting is a good way to restore your soul, you may be confused by the traditional rabbinic definition of *work*. Because some of these activities may not feel like work, you may wonder where the definition of *work* comes from.

The rabbinic definition of work is derived from the story of the building of God's tabernacle. After the exodus from Egypt, when the Children of Israel are wandering in the desert, they build a tabernacle for God. The Torah records all the detailed instructions that they are given on how to build it (Exodus 25:1–40:38). The rabbis analyzed and categorized all the tabernacle instructions into a list of thirty-nine different activities. The thirty-nine activities used in building the tabernacle form the basis of the traditional Jewish legal definition of work. They include planting, sewing, lighting a fire, hitting with a hammer (usually understood as "giving the finishing touch" to something), and so on.[13] In traditional Shabbat observance, any activity that falls into one of these thirty-nine categories is *work* and therefore cannot be done on Shabbat.

Immediately after Moses receives the instructions on how to build the tabernacle, God reminds him that no one is to work on Shabbat. "But keep My Shabbats, for it is a sign between Me and you for all of your generations, to know that I, YHVH, make you holy" (Exodus 31:13). Rashi interprets the word *but* in the passage to mean "But do not put off Shabbat in your eager enthusiasm for the work of building the tabernacle."[14] Even building God's holy tabernacle does not take precedence over Shabbat resting!

The connection between building God's home and resting on Shabbat—preserved in the laws of Shabbat in great detail—is there as a reminder that, even if one is doing the holiest work in the world, even building a home for God, one needs to stop and rest on Shabbat. The only exception to this is if one needs to save a life.

When one stops working, one frees oneself to focus on the positive activities for Shabbat, such as lighting candles, hearing the weekly Torah portion, praying, eating with friends and family, and saying special Shabbat blessings. Stopping work and filling one's life with light, wisdom, prayer, food, friends, family, and blessings is a way to rest that restores the soul.

## Mystical Resting

According to Sfat Emet, rest is found at your root. "There is no exertion when a person cleaves to his root, which is the place where there is rest."[15] What and where is your root?

Consider for a moment the roots of a tree. Through its roots, a tree draws the vitality it needs from deep in the earth into the very edges of its highest leaves. Sfat Emet teaches that people have a root as well. Like the root of a tree that is connected to the sustaining vitality of the earth, the root of a person is connected to the sustaining vitality of God. We draw our vital energy through our roots. The more one cleaves to one's root, the more vitality one can draw from God.

Sfat Emet teaches that your root is within you. He often calls it the inner point. Cleaving to your inner point is an essential mystical idea and practice. Jewish mystics simply call it *d'vekút* (cleaving). According to Sfat Emet, connecting and cleaving to your inner point not only leads you to the most desirable resting place, it leads you to the deepest and most intimate knowledge, the knowledge of God.[16]

Just as the soul and resting are inseparable, so are resting and God. "Your children will recognize and know in the most intimate way that their rest comes from You."[17] The complete rest of love, generosity, truth, faith, peace, serenity, quiet, and security is at your root and comes from God.

## Your Root and the Days of the Week

Sometimes during the week, the gateway to your root is closed, but on Shabbat, the gateway opens and your root is revealed. By cleaving to one's root on Shabbat, one receives vital energy not only for Shabbat but also for all the days of the week. "This is the essential meaning of Shabbat, to cleave to the root of life through which all the days of the week are blessed."[18]

Shabbat wakes up the root of all things, because Shabbat connects this world to the root of vital life energy of the upper worlds. The more one connects to one's root on Shabbat, the more one can discover it even in the days of the week.[19] In other words, the more you rest on Shabbat, the more restful your working week will be.

## The Strength to Stop

The fourth commandment says to "work for six days and do *all* your work" (Exodus 20:9). Rashi detects a problem with being commanded to do *all* of our work. Who actually completes all of their work? In Jewish tradition, even God, in the creation of heaven and earth, did not complete all of the work of creation. Recognizing the problem that no one ever completes all of their work, Rashi explains the passage: "When the seventh day comes it should be in your eyes *as if* you have done all of your work. You should not even think about your work."[20] In other words, even though all of your work is not done by the time Shabbat arrives, you should think and act *as if* it is done.

It takes great willpower, great strength of mind not only to stop working but also to stop thinking about your work. In Jerusalem on Friday evenings, at the sunset hour when white stones are illuminated with the golden rays of the setting sun, you can hear this sweet song in one of the synagogues: "If only I had the strength, I would go to the marketplace and cry out: Today is Shabbat, Oy, today is Shabbat for God." In an overly materialist world, where stores never close and cell phones never stop ringing, it takes strength to stop and make time for the soul.

## Reminder of Freedom

Shabbat is called a reminder that we have left Egypt.[21] In Egypt, we were slaves. We worked all the time. Tradition teaches that the slavery in Egypt began when Pharaoh convinced us to work on Shabbat. His taskmasters called us lazy for wanting to rest. Do you have taskmasters inside you that do not let you rest?

Work itself is not a problem. Work is good. We are even commanded to work. Sfat Emet teaches that wherever you see Shabbat mentioned in the Torah, you see the six days of work mentioned as well.[22] For example: "You should work for six days and do all your work. And the seventh day is Shabbat for YHVH your God" (Exodus 20:9, 10). Working and resting complement and complete each other, like a well-matched couple. Sfat Emet describes the six days of the week as the wax for the candle that we light on Shabbat.[23] The work you do transforms and ascends to its true spiritual stature on Shabbat. If you do not work, there is no wax, no candle to light. If you only work, you are an unlit candle.

Working is only a problem when you never stop, when you do not remember that "the seventh day is Shabbat" (Exodus 20:10). If you cannot stop what you are doing, then you are a slave to your work. Learning to act and feel and even think as if all your work is done can transform you from being a slave to your work to being free. Let every Shabbat remind you that you are free. You can stop working. You are allowed to rest.

According to Rabbi Heschel, "Civilization is on trial. Its future will depend upon how much of the Shabbat will penetrate its spirit."[24]

## Yoga Practice for Remembering to Rest

Make some time to stop working now. Pause and breathe. In these restorative postures, connect and cleave inward to your root, and feel the delight of resting.

# Opening Meditation

Sit on a firm folded blanket with your buttocks on the blanket and your feet on the floor. Cross your legs, and release the tops of your thighs down. Pull the flesh of your buttocks out to the sides and diagonally back. Press your sitz bones into your blanket, and on an inhalation, extend your spine up through the crown of your head. Rest your hands on your knees (see Chapter One, Photo 1.1).

Gently close your eyes. Relax your face. Turn your gaze inward. Soften inside. Spend a few moments observing your breath. Feel your breath naturally coming in and going out.

Affirm to yourself that, during the following postures, you will not busy yourself thinking about things you need to do. Let go of thinking about what you were doing before you began your practice. Let go of thinking about what you need to do when you finish your practice.

Do not be hard on yourself when busy thoughts appear. Each time they vie for your attention, gently release them; bring your awareness back to your breath and to the sensations of your body.

Feel your awareness moving inward. Establish a connection to a realm of quiet and rest within you. Open your eyes.

---

### RESTORATIVE POSTURES AND THE RELAXATION POSTURE

In these restorative postures, take time to set yourself up in each posture with the support you need. Once you are set up comfortably in a posture, consciously let go of any effort or exertion.

For these postures, it will be helpful to have several firm blankets and a bolster. If you do not have a bolster you can use more firm blankets instead. These props help make the postures more restful and restorative.

The Relaxation Posture that is taught at the end of this chapter is traditionally practiced at the end of every yoga session. Although every chapter in this book ends with a relaxing posture, you may want to add this classic Relaxation Posture as well.

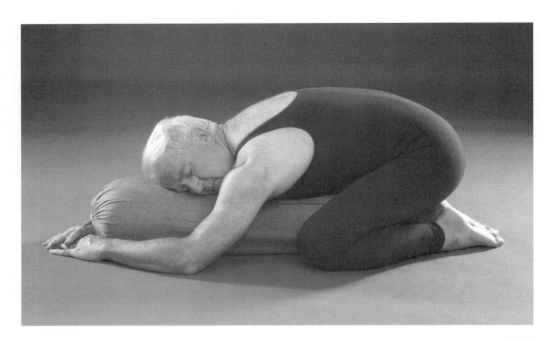

**Photo 39.1**

# Supported Extended Child Posture

Sit on your heels, and place a bolster lengthwise in front of you. Take your knees out a little wider than your hips and bring the bolster in close to you, between your thighs.

Bend forward and rest your whole torso on the bolster, with your arms folded around the top end of the bolster. Keep your hips on your heels, and lengthen your spine forward along the bolster. Turn your head to one side (Photo 39.1). Feel the support of the bolster under you, and let go.

Alternatively, you can place a blanket on the end of the bolster and rest your forehead and folded arms up on the blanket (Photo 39.2). This way, your neck stays in alignment with your spine.

If you need more height in order to be comfortable, place a folded blanket lengthwise on the bolster. If your hips are up off your heels, place a folded blanket on top of your calves.

Relax your face and eyes. Quiet yourself inside. Give yourself permission to rest your active mind and body. Let thoughts float away and feel tensions melt.

Rest here for a few minutes. Then if your head is turned to one side, slowly turn your head to the second side and continue resting a few more minutes.

    To release, press your hands into the floor, and sit upright.

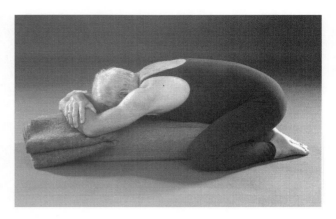

**Photo 39.2**

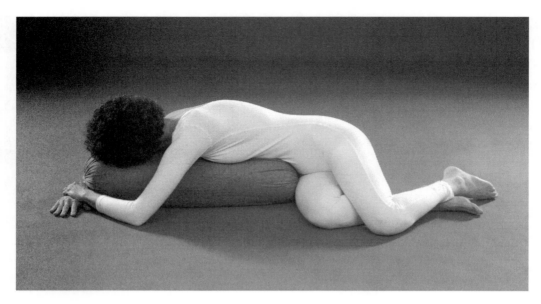

**Photo 40.1**

# Resting Side Twist

Sit on your buttocks with your knees bent and your feet pointing behind you on your left side. Place a bolster lengthwise out from your right hip.

Inhale and lengthen your spine. Exhale and twist your torso from left to right so that the front of your torso faces your bolster. With your torso gently twisted, lay the front of your torso over the bolster, and rest on the left side of your face. If your neck feels strained, rest on the right side of your face. Hug your arms around the front of the bolster (Photo 40.1).

Soften and close your eyes. Relax your belly. Notice whether you feel tension anywhere or whether you are using effort to hold yourself up, and let it go. Allow yourself to be in this posture for several minutes. Let this twist wring tensions out of your spine. Let yourself unwind.

To release, press your hands gently into the floor and come up to sitting. Open your eyes. Turn your torso to face forward, and then repeat the posture on the other side.

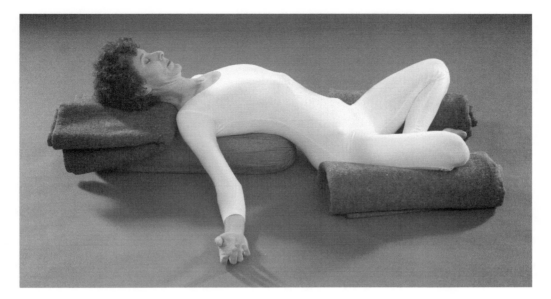

**Photo 41.1**

# Supported Fish Posture

Sit cross-legged on the floor. Place a bolster lengthwise behind your buttocks, with a folded blanket for your head on top of the end of the bolster. Place a rolled blanket beside you on both sides of your thighs.

On an inhalation, lengthen your spine. Exhale and recline halfway back, using your hands for support. Lift your buttocks slightly, and move your tailbone and buttocks toward your knees; then lower your buttocks back down. Lengthen your spine away from your legs, and lift your chest.

Rest the back of your trunk on your bolster with your head and neck supported by your blanket, so that your forehead is higher than your chin. Place the rolled blankets underneath your thighs and knees, high enough to support your legs. If you feel strain in your lower back, move your tailbone and buttocks more toward your knees and lengthen your spine away from your legs. Relax your arms down by your sides, palms facing up, fingers curled (Photo 41.1).

Relax your eyes, and be attentive to your inner world. Notice your inhalations and your exhalations. Notice the still moment between breaths. Quiet your mind. Relax your muscles.

Rest here for a few minutes. Let tension go with each outgoing breath. Find your root of rest, the place beyond any turmoil and tension.

To come out of this posture, use your hands to draw your knees back together. Roll to your right side, and lie in the fetal position for a few breaths. Press your hands into the floor, and come back to sitting.

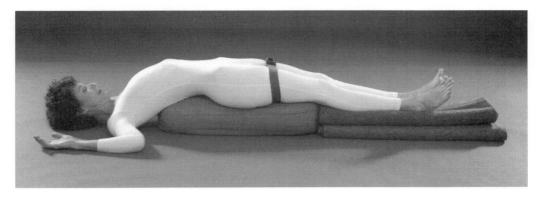

**Photo 42.1**

# Supported Bridge Posture

For this posture, you will need (1) two bolsters or a bolster and several folded blankets and (2) a belt. Set up your bolsters, or bolster and folded blankets, end to end so that they are long enough for you to lie on lengthwise and are all the same height.

Sit in Staff Posture (see Chapter Three, Photo 15.1) on your bolster or blankets with your back about two feet from the end. Secure a belt firmly around the middle of your thighs to hold your legs together.

On an inhalation, lengthen your spine. Lift your chest and lean back onto your elbows. Lower yourself down and back, draping your middle and upper back over the end of the bolster. Bring the back of your neck and head and the tops of your shoulders down onto the floor.

Bring your arms out to your sides, elbows bent, palms facing up, on either side of your head. Relax the back of your neck (Photo 42.1). Never turn your head from side to side in this posture.

Straighten your legs, and press out through your heels and the balls of your feet. Then relax your legs. Let the belt hold your legs so that you can completely let go of any effort to keep them together.

Feel the bolsters under you, supporting your back and your opening heart. Soften your eyes. Relax all the muscles in your face. Relax your lips and your tongue. Let the bolsters completely support your body.

Look inward to your heart and soul. Feel your ribs and diaphragm expanding and broadening, making more space for extra breath to come into your lungs.

Rest in this posture for several minutes. Slow down and relax your breath. Observe your breath coming in and going out. See how your breath quiets your mind and relaxes your body. Delight in the sensations of soulful resting.

To release, bend your knees and loosen your belt. Roll slowly off the bolster to your right side. Rest on your side for a few breaths. Then press your hands into the floor to come up to sitting.

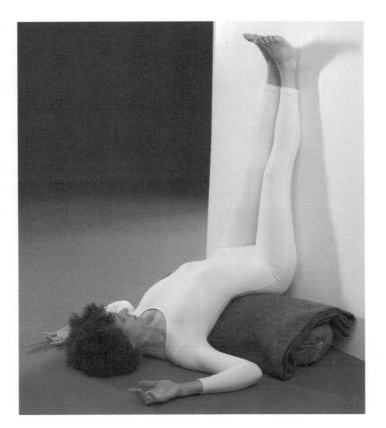

# Gentle Inversion Posture

Place a bolster parallel to and a few inches away from a wall. Sit on the edge of the bolster, with your left hip and shoulder toward the wall, knees bent (Photo 43.1).

Place your right hand on the floor in front of the middle of the bolster. Lift your hips up, and place your outer right hip on the bolster. Bring your left hip over your right, and move your buttocks close to the wall.

Lower down onto your right elbow, then your right shoulder, keeping your hips on the bolster (Photo 43.2).

Roll onto your back, bringing your shoulders and back of your head to the floor and both buttocks evenly against the wall.

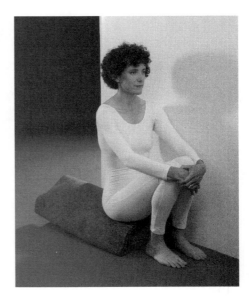

**Photo 43.1**

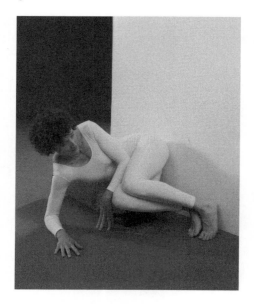

**Photo 43.2**

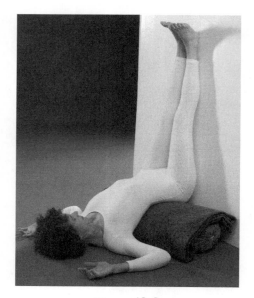

**Photo 43.3**

Adjust the bolster by pulling it underneath your back ribs and lower back so that it supports an opening in your chest.

Move your shoulder blades down toward your waist and roll the tops of your shoulders down toward the floor. Stretch your legs up the wall and press them back toward the wall.

Bring your arms out to your sides, elbows bent, palms facing up, on either side of your head (Photo 43.3). Close your eyes, and turn your attention inward. Relax in this posture for several minutes. Let gravity draw you deep into your root of rest.

To release, bend your knees and place your feet on the wall. Push yourself back off your bolster, and rest on your back. Roll to your side, and lie in fetal position for a few breaths, then open your eyes. Press your hands into the floor to come up to sitting.

# Glossary

THE GLOSSARY PRESENTS SOME JEWISH BACKGROUND for the text of *Torah Yoga*. This background is not necessary for understanding the rest of the book. The *Encyclopaedia Judaica* has been an important source for the information presented here.

**Ari**  Rabbi Isaac ben Solomon Luria (1534–1572), known by his contemporaries as Rabbi Isaac Ashkenazi, or Rabbi Isaac Ashkenazi Luria, or simply as de Luria, is usually called the *Ari* (lion). Although it is often said that one may not study Kabbalah until one is at least forty years old, the Ari died at age thirty-nine as perhaps the greatest Kabbalist ever. He was born in Jerusalem, but after his father died while he was still a boy, his mother took him to Egypt to live. The last few years of his short life, he returned to live in Sefad, Israel, marking it as the center of Kabbalistic knowledge at its peak. He published only one short work himself, a commentary on a short section of the *Zohar* (splendor), thus his work is known mostly from the writings of his disciples.

**Baal Shem Tov**  Israel ben Eliezer (c. 1700–1760), known as the Baal Shem Tov (Master of the Good Name) and as the Besht (acronym of Baal Shem Tov), was the charismatic founder of the Hasidic movement. He was an itinerant teacher, storyteller, and miracle worker in Poland, which for a thousand years was the center of the Eastern European Jewish community. He did not publish anything himself; all the stories about him and those attributed to him are due to the writings of his many famous disciples. His teachings emphasized praying for individual salvation, mystical cleaving to God, and the ideal of the *tsaddik* (righteous one, or saint).

**Gemara**  See Talmud.

**Haggadah**   This very old compilation of sacred texts on the exodus from Egypt is considered a sacred text in its own right. Used on the first night of Passover as the basic order of service for that night and its festive meal, it retells the exodus in its own fashion—without mentioning the name of Moses, for example—and encourages extensive questioning and discussion of every aspect of the exodus and freedom. Those who question and discuss the most—even continuing until the next morning—are the most praiseworthy.

**Hasidim**   Followers of the Baal Shem Tov and his disciples are known as Hasidim. The name literally means "pious ones." Hasidism was, and still is, a diverse movement with many different and even contradictory characteristics. For some Hasidim, joy and ecstasy are central aspects of prayer and life. Others emphasize fasting and other ascetic practices. A Rebbe, usually considered a *tsaddik* (righteous person) by his followers, is the spiritual leader of a Hasidic community. Many such communities are named after the place where they originally began, such as the Satmar (Rumania), Gur (Poland), Lubavich (Russia), Karlin (Lithuania), and so on.

**Ibn Ezra**   Abraham Ibn Ezra (1089–1164) was born in Tudela, Spain. From 1140 until his death, he was a wandering poet, teacher, and physician, traveling mostly in Italy and France. Tradition says he spent the last few years of his life in Israel. He is known as the father of biblical criticism.

**Kabbalah**   Kabbalah means "receiving." It is esoteric, mystical, hidden Jewish wisdom that, traditionally, students receive directly from their teacher. Although it has been an aspect of study for a select few since the first century, it became more widely known in the early middle ages. Today it is a popular subject for many.

**Maimonides**   Moses ben Maimon (1135–1204), known as the Rambam, (RMBM, an acronym for Rabbi Moses Ben Maimon), was the leading rabbinic authority, codifier, philosopher, and royal physician of his generation. He was born in Cordova, Spain.

**Malbim**   Meir Loeb Ben Yehiel Michael (1809–1879), born in Volhynia, Poland, is known as the Malbim (based on the acronym formed by his name, MLBYM). He is famous for his complete commentaries on the Tanach, published from 1860 to 1876.

**Midrash**   The word *Midrash* itself means "study, explanation, interpretation." The Midrash is the collective name for a large body of midrashic literature— literature that gives legal or homiletic interpretations of the Torah. Examples of Midrash include *Midrash Rabba* (great midrash), and *Yalkut Shimoni* (Simon's anthology).

**Mishnah**    See Talmud.

**Rabbeinu Bachya**    Bachya ben Asher ben Chlava, a thirteenth-century teacher and Kabbalist, is known for his commentary on the Torah, written in 1291.

**Rabbi Abraham Joshua Heschel**    Rabbi Heschel (1907–1972) was one of the most influential U.S. Jewish thinkers of the twentieth century. He was born in Germany and came to the United States in 1940. He was a teacher, scholar, mystic, philosopher, and prolific writer. His books include *The Sabbath, Man Is Not Alone,* and *God in Search of Man.*

**Rabbi Akiva**    was a first century sage who only began to study Torah later in life. He is considered to be one of the greatest Torah scholars and teachers throughout Jewish history.

**Rabbi Bunem**    Simcha Bunem (1765–1827) was the *tsaddik* (righteous person) of the Hasidic community in Pshiskha, Poland.

**Rabbi Eliezer**    Eliezer ben Hyrcanus was known as Eliezer the Great or simply as Rabbi Eliezer. He lived in Israel in the early second century and was one of the greatest Talmudic sages.

**Rashi**    Rabbi Shlomo ben Isaac (1040–1105), known by the acronym Rashi (RShI), was born and lived in Troyes, France. His commentaries on Torah and Talmud are considered as one of the indispensable starting points for all serious students of Torah and Talmud. As he stated explicitly, his goal was to make clear the literal meaning of the text. To do this, he drew on earlier rabbinic sources and his own extensive knowledge of Hebrew grammar. Because he sometimes translated into his contemporary French, his works are primary source material for linguistic students of Old French.

**Rav Kook**    Rabbi Abraham Isaac Kook (1865–1935), born in Latvia, was an ardent Zionist. As Rav is the Hebrew word for rabbi, he is often called Rav Kook. He was the first Ashkenazi Chief Rabbi of Israel in the 1930s. Rav Kook was a scholar, mystic, and prolific poetic writer. His works include *Orót haKódesh* (lights of holiness), *Orót* (lights), and *Orót haTshuváh* (lights of repentance).

**Resh Lakish**    Rabbi Shimon ben Lakish was a third-century rabbi who was born and lived in Israel, around Tiberias.

***Sfat Emet***    *Sfat Emet* (language of truth) is the name of the collected writings of Rabbi Judah Aryeh Leib Alter (1847–1905). The name *Sfat Emet* is commonly used to refer to Rabbi Alter himself as well. Rabbi Alter was the third Rebbe of the Hasidim of Gur, Poland. After 1939, the Hasidim of Gur relocated to Jerusalem, Israel, where they are a vibrant community to this day.

**Shabbat**　Shabbat is the Jewish Sabbath. It begins Friday evening a little before sunset and continues until Saturday well after sunset (until one can see three stars on a clear night). All Jewish days start in the evening, based on the example given in Genesis 1:5, "and there was evening, and there was morning, one day." Shabbat, roughly corresponding to Saturday, is the only day of the week in Hebrew that actually has its own name. Sunday, Monday, Tuesday, Wednesday, Thursday, and Friday (named respectively after the sun, the moon, and the Norse mythological deities Tewi, Woden, Thor, and Frigga) are called in Hebrew First Day, Second Day, Third Day, Fourth Day, Fifth Day, and Sixth Day (toward Shabbat is understood).

*Shulchan Aruch*　(The Prepared Table) A codification of Jewish law written by Joseph Caro in the sixteenth century in Italy.

**Talmud**　There are actually two: the Babylonian Talmud and the Jerusalem Talmud. They were compiled roughly in parallel in Babylonia (modern Iraq) and Israel after the destruction of the second Temple. The Jerusalem Talmud was "finished" earlier (c. 400 CE) than the Babylonian Talmud (c. 499 CE). They both contain the Mishnah and Gemara. The Mishnah contains concise statements of oral law; the Gemara contains further discussion of points in the Mishnah. The Talmud also contains *Aggada* (stories) that are historical, biographical, philosophical, and mystical in nature.

**Tanach**　*Tanach* is an acronym for *Torah* (Teaching), *Nevi'im* (Prophets), and *Ketuvim* (Writings), the three parts of the Jewish Bible.

**Torah**　The Torah, strictly speaking, includes only the five books of Moses (the Pentateuch: Genesis, Exodus, Leviticus, Numbers, and Deuteronomy). Special Hebrew scribes manually write out copies of the Torah on a single parchment scroll. These scrolls, dressed and decorated, are kept in the *aron kodesh* (holy cabinet) of synagogues. Each week in traditional synagogues, a portion of the Torah is chanted to the congregation so that over a year they hear the entire scroll. An extensive definition of the word Torah is given in the Introduction.

*Zohar*　The *Zohar* (Splendor) is the primary text of Jewish mysticism. It is divided into five books. Its putative author is Shimon bar Yochai. Some scholars attribute it to Moses ben Shem Tov de Leon (d. 1305).

# Notes

Prayers in the book were translated from the Hebrew by the author. Readers interested in more complete versions of the prayers can refer to *The Complete Artscroll Siddur-Sefard* (Brooklyn, N.Y.: Mesorah Publications, 1985), or to other traditional Siddurim (prayer books).

## Introduction

1. Rashi on Deuteronomy 33:2.

2. B.K.S. Iyengar quoted in *Yoga Rahasya,* 2003, *10*(2), p. 10.

3. Reproduction of talk with Geeta S. Iyengar, "Religious and Lingual Barriers to Yoga," *Yoga Rahasya,* 2003, *10*(2), p. 9.

4. Ibn Ezra on Exodus 25:40.

5. B.K.S. Iyengar, *Yoga: The Path to Holistic Health* (London: Dorling Kindersley, 2001), p. 14.

6. B.K.S. Iyengar, *Yoga: The Path to Holistic Health* (London.: Dorling Kindersley 2001), p. 14.

7. *Ethics of the Fathers* 5:26.

8. *Midrash Rabba,* Genesis 1:1.

9. Daniel C. Matt, trans. and ed., *Zohar: The Book of Enlightenment* (Mahwah, N.J.: Paulist Press, 1983), pp. 206–207, summarizing *Zohar* 3:152a.

10. Daily Prayer Book, Evening Service, second blessing before the Shma (Hear, oh Israel . . .).

11. Schneur Zalman of Liadi, *Sha'ar ha-Yihud ve-ha-Emunah* (The Gate of Unity and Faith) (Brooklyn, N.Y.: Kehot Publication Society, 1981), p. 152.

## Using This Book

1. *Ethics of the Fathers* 6:6.

# Chapter One: The Hidden Light

1. Ashlag, Yehuda. *Sefer Hahakdamot* (The Book of Introductions) Introduction to the Zohar (New York: Kabbalah Publishing, 1986).

2. Malbim on Song of Songs, Chapter 8 HeCharash VeHamasger (The Craftsman and the Locksmith).

3. Malbim on Psalms 8:7.

4. Abraham Isaac Kook, *Chadarav* (His Room) (Israel: Reoot Publishers, 1997), p. 29.

5. Babylonian Talmud, *Chaggigah* 12a.

6. *Zohar* 1:20a, 2:137a, 2:166b; Daniel C. Matt, trans. and ed., *Zohar: The Book of Enlightenment* (Mahwah, N.J.: Paulist Press, 1983), p. 210.

7. Yehudah Ashlag. *Sefer Hahakdamot* (The Book of Introductions) Introduction to the Zohar (New York: Kabbalah Publishing, 1986).

8. *Yalkut Shimoni* 1:4 on Genesis.

9. Aryeh Kaplan, *The Bahir Illumination* (York Beach, Maine: Samuel Weiser, 1979), pp. xxi–xxv.

10. *Rabba Genesis* 6:3, for example.

11. Babylonian Talmud, *Chaggigah* 12a.

12. *Zohar* 1:47a, 2:20b, 3:88a; Daniel C. Matt, trans. and ed., *Zohar: The Book of Enlightenment* (Mahwah, N.J.: Paulist Press, 1983), p. 211.

13. Babylonian Talmud, *Chaggigah* 12a.

14. Maimonides, *Hilchot Tshuvah* 5:2.

15. Daniel C.Matt, trans. and ed., *Zohar: The Book of Enlightenment* (Mahwah, N.J.: Paulist Press, 1983), p. 214.

16. Rashi on Exodus 2:2.

17. Sfat Emet on Genesis, p. 204.

# Chapter Two: Constant Renewal

1. Sfat Emet on Genesis, p. 85.

2. Sfat Emet on Genesis, p. 83.

3. Statement attributed to Heraclitus.

4. Sfat Emet on Genesis, p. 200.

5. Any traditional Daily, Shabbat, or Festival Prayer Book, Morning Service, first blessing before the Shma (Hear, oh Israel . . .).

6. Abraham Isaac Kook, *Orot Hakodesh* (Lights of Holiness), Vol. 2 (Jerusalem: The Rav Kook Institute, 1963), p. 517.

7. Sfat Emet on Genesis, p. 200.

8. Sfat Emet on Leviticus, p. 13.

9. Sfat Emet on Leviticus, p. 16.

10. Abraham Isaac Kook, *Orot Hakodesh* (Lights of Holiness), Vol. 2 (Jerusalem: The Rav Kook Institute, 1963), p. 165.

## Chapter Three: Leaving Egypt

1. Commentary in *The Wine of Torah, Haggadah.*

2. Abraham Isaac Kook, *Chadarav* (His Room) (Israel: Reoot Publishers, 1997), p. 39.

3. Mishnah, *Brachot* 1:5. These two Mishnaic teachings are also in the Haggadah.

4. Sfat Emet on Exodus, p. 55.

5. Sfat Emet on Exodus, p. 25.

6. Any traditional Daily, Shabbat, or Festival Prayer Book, Morning and Evening Services, third paragraph of the Shma (Hear, oh Israel . . .).

7. Any traditional Shabbat or Festival Prayer Book, Kiddush (Sanctification), wine blessing.

8. See Aryeh Kaplan. *Waters of Eden: The Mystery of the Mikveh* (New York: NCSY Union of Orthodox Jewish Congregations of America, 1976).

## Chapter Four: The Essential Self

1. Rashi on Genesis 3:9.

2. Abraham Isaac Kook, *Orot Hakodesh* (Lights of Holiness), Vol. 3 (Jerusalem: The Rav Kook Institute, 1963), p. 140.

3. *Ethics of the Fathers* 1:16.

4. *Ethics of the Fathers* 1:15.

5. *Zohar* 1:78a; Daniel C. Matt, *The Essential Kabbalah: The Heart of Jewish Mysticism* (San Francisco: HarperSanFrancisco, 1996), p. 127.

6. Lawrence Kushner, *God Was in This Place and I, I Did Not Know* (Woodstock, N.Y.: Jewish Lights Publishing, 1991).

7. Abraham Isaac Kook, *Orot Hakodesh* (Lights of Holiness) Vol.3 (Jerusalem: The Rav Kook Institute, 1963), p. 140.

8. Abraham Isaac Kook, *Orot Hakodesh* (Lights of Holiness) Vol.3 (Jerusalem: The Rav Kook Institute, 1963), p. 140.

9. Babylonian Talmud, Tractate Chulin 60:2 and Rashi on Genesis 1:16.

10. Abraham Isaac Kook, *Orot Hakodesh* (Lights of Holiness) Vol.3 (Jerusalem: The Rav Kook Institute, 1963), p. 130.

11. Abraham Isaac Kook, *Orot Hakodesh* (Lights of Holiness) Vol.3 (Jerusalem: The Rav Kook Institute, 1963), p. 175.

12. Abraham Isaac Kook, *Orot Hakodesh* (Lights of Holiness) Vol.3 (Jerusalem: The Rav Kook Institute, 1963), p. 141.

13. Abraham Isaac Kook, *Orot Hakodesh* (Lights of Holiness) Vol.3 (Jerusalem: The Rav Kook Institute, 1963), p. 141.

# Chapter Five: Body Prayer and Alignment

1. Martin Buber, *Or Haganuz* (The Hidden Light) (Tel Aviv: Schocken, 1979).

2. Sfat Emet.

3. Any traditional Shabbat or Festival Prayer Book, Morning Service, excerpt from the Nishmat Kol Chai (Breath of Every Living Thing) prayer [words in bold are D. Bloomfield's emphasis].

4. Abraham Isaac Kook, *Olat Reayah* (The Offering of Rabbi Abraham Isaac HaCohen Kook), Vol. 1 (Jerusalem: The Rav Kook Institute), p. 11.

5. Abraham Isaac Kook, *Olat Reayah* (The Offering of Rabbi Abraham Isaac HaCohen Kook), Vol. 1 (Jerusalem: The Rav Kook Institute), p. 73.

6. Abraham Isaac Kook, *Olat Reayah* (The Offering of Rabbi Abraham Isaac HaCohen Kook), Vol. 1 (Jerusalem: The Rav Kook Institute), p. 73.

7. Abraham Isaac Kook, *Olat Reayah* (The Offering of Rabbi Abraham Isaac HaCohen Kook), Vol. 1 (Jerusalem: The Rav Kook Institute), p. 73.

8. Babylonian Talmud, *Brachot* 60b.

9. Abraham Isaac Kook, *Olat Reayah* (The Offering of Rabbi Abraham Isaac HaCohen Kook), Vol. 1 (Jerusalem: The Rav Kook Institute), p. 73.

10. Babylonian Talmud, *Brachot* 12a.

11. Babylonian Talmud, Menachot 43b.

# Chapter Six: Daily Satisfaction

1. Rashi on Exodus 16:13.

2. *Midrash Rabba,* Exodus 24:1.

3. Rabbeinu Bachya on Exodus 34:28.

4. Mathew Fox, lecture at Elat Chayyim Jewish Retreat Center, Woodstock, New York, July 1991.

5. Amy Waldman, "For Yoga Guru, Reaching Perfection Is a Stretch," *New York Times,* Dec. 14, 2002, p. A4.

6. Kli Yakar on Exodus 16:15.

7. Any traditional Prayer Book.

8. *The Pentateuch and Haftorahs Hebrew Text, English Translation and Commentary,* 2nd edition, Dr. J. H. Hertz, ed. (London: Soncino Press, 1978), p. 276.

9. Sforno on Exodus 16:16.

10. Rashi on Exodus 16:17.

11. Rabbeinu Bachyai on Exodus 34:28.

12. Any traditional Prayer Book.

13. Any traditional Shabbat or Festival Prayer Book, Morning, Afternoon, and Evening Service, excerpt from the Amidah (Standing) prayer.

14. Any traditional Daily, Shabbat, or Festival Prayer Book, Morning, Afternoon, and Evening Service, excerpt from the Ashrei (Happy are they . . .) prayer.

## Chapter Seven: Remembering to Rest

1. *Midrash Rabba,* Genesis 46.2.

2. *The Pentateuch and Haftorahs Hebrew Text, English Translation and Commentary,* 2nd edition, Dr. J. H. Hertz, ed. (London: Soncino Press, 1978), p. 6.

3. B.K.S. Iyengar, *Yoga: The Path to Holistic Health,* Yoga Sutra 11.47 (London: Dorling Kindersley, 2001), p. 17.

4. Francis Brown, S. R. Driver, and C. A. Briggs, *Hebrew and English Lexicon of the Old Testament* (Oxford: Clarendon Press, 1959), p. 661.

5. Mitsudat Tsion on II Samuel 16:14.

6. Everett Fox, *The Five Books of Moses—Genesis, Exodus, Leviticus, Numbers, Deuteronomy: A New Translation with Introduction, Commentary, and Notes by Everett Fox* (New York: Schocken Books, 1995), p. 436.

7. Or HaChayim on Genesis 2:2.

8. Babylonian Talmud, *Baitza* 16a.

9. Abraham Joshua Heschel, *Man Is Not Alone* (New York: Noon Day Press, 1997), p. 191 (Originally Published 1951 by Farrar, Straus and Giroux).

10. Abraham Isaac Kook, *Chadarav* (His Room) (Israel: Reoot Publishers, 1997), pp. 35, 39, 40.

11. Any traditional Shabbat Prayer Book, Additional Morning Service, excerpt from the Amidah (Standing) prayer.

12. Any traditional Shabbat Prayer Book, Afternoon Service, excerpt from the Amidah (Standing) prayer.

13. Mishnah, *Shabbat* 7:2.

14. Rashi on Exodus 31:13.

15. Sfat Emet on Genesis, p. 20.

16. Sfat Emet on Exodus, p. 197.

17. Any traditional Shabbat Prayer Book, Afternoon Service, excerpt from the Amidah (Standing) prayer.

18. Sfat Emet on Exodus, p. 197.

19. Sfat Emet on Exodus, p. 198.

20. Rashi on Exodus 20:9.

21. Any traditional Shabbat or Festival Prayer Book, Kiddush (Sanctification) wine blessing.

22. Sfat Emet on Exodus, p. 104.

23. Sfat Emet.

24. Abraham Joshua Heschel, *God in Search of Man* (New York: Farrar, Straus & Cudahy, 1955), p. 418.

# Annotated Yoga Bibliography

T HE FOLLOWING IS A LIST of books and videos that I have
found to be particularly helpful, insightful, and inspirational for
my yoga practice.

## Yoga Books

Farhi, D., *Yoga Mind, Body and Spirit: A Return to Wholeness.* New York: Henry
Holt, 2000.

This is a holistic approach to yoga, viewed through the lens of the organic,
nervous, cellular, musculoskeletal, and other systems of the body.

Iyengar, B.K.S. *Yoga, the Path to Holistic Health.* New York: Dorling Kindersley,
2001.

The author presents a wide range of yoga postures and gives extensive information about associated health benefits and precautions.

Iyengar, G. *Yoga, a Gem for Women.* Spokane, Wash.: Timeless Books, 1990.

This book presents traditional yoga postures and highlights benefits and
special instructions for women in all stages of life.

Schiffmann, E. *Yoga, the Spirit and Practice of Moving into Stillness.* New York:
Simon & Schuster, 1996.

This personal, spiritual approach to yoga teaches you to how to practice postures at the level that is right for you.

Silva, M., and Mehta, S. *Yoga the Iyengar Way.* New York: Knopf, 1996.

Silva and Mehta give clear and detailed instructions for most of the fundamental yoga postures. B.K.S. Iyengar wrote the foreword.

## Yoga Videos

MacGraw, A. *Ali MacGraw Yoga Mind and Body.* Burbank: Warner Home Video, 1994.

This video offers an intermediate-level yoga practice, with inspirational music and beautiful choreography.

Walden, P. *Yoga Journal's Yoga for Beginners.* Gaiam, 1996.

Walden, one of today's leading Iyengar teachers, offers a wide range of clearly described beginning yoga postures.

Wenig, M. *YogaKids, an Easy, Fun-filled Adventure.* Gaiam, 1996.

This is a creative and playful yoga practice for children, with lots of animals and beautiful scenery.

# The Author

DIANE BLOOMFIELD is the creator of Torah Yoga and has been developing this integrative approach to Jewish wisdom since the early 1990s. She teaches Torah Yoga workshops and classes throughout North America, Western Europe, and Israel.

She has been studying Torah for many years—in traditional yeshivas, with private teachers, and on her own. In her private Torah study, she concentrates on the teachings of Sfat Emet, a Hasidic master, and Rav Kook, the visionary first Chief Rabbi of Israel.

The author began her yoga studies at the Kripalu Institute in Massachusetts and has continued to train with teachers spanning a wide range of yoga styles such as Bikram and Iyengar. She is a certified Phoenix Rising yoga therapist.

The author has lived primarily in Israel since 1984. Currently, she and her husband and daughter are living in St. Paul, Minnesota.

Bloomfield, Diane,
1959-

Torah yoga.

| DATE | | | |
|---|---|---|---|
| | | | |
| | | | |
| | | | |
| | | | |
| | | | |
| | | | |
| | | | |
| | | | |
| | | | |
| | | | |
| | | | |
| | | | |
| | | | |

BAKER & TAYLOR